ANTHROPOSOPHICAL THERAPEUTIC SPEECH

ANTHROPOSOPHICAL THERAPEUTIC SPEECH

Barbara Denjean-von Stryk
Dietrich von Bonin

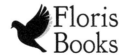

Floris
Books

Contents

Part Two: The Practice of Therapeutic Speech

case examples in the manuscript and offering suggestions with medical terminology; Anna Phillips, for translating the untranslatable German words and phrases and having them make sense in the English; Brenda Ratcliffe, for creating English equivalents to the many verses and pinpointing English poetry to match the original German; and the many others who have read through the draft manuscript and offered valuable suggestions.

May this book find its way into many cross-professional hands in addition to those practising Anthroposophical Therapeutic Speech. It will serve to broaden the contemporary concepts of speech and voice therapy.

Donald Phillips
Aberdeen, Scotland

Foreword to the German edition

This book was originally published in German as the volume of a four-volume documentation of anthroposophic art therapy. It was the result of an international co-operation that took place over ten years, between 1989 and 1998. More than one hundred and twenty art therapists from Germany, Great Britain, Finland, the Netherlands, Switzerland, Italy, Norway, France and Austria worked together in nine study groups with several doctors to collect and exchange their therapeutic experience and theoretical approaches from their respective artistic fields. It was the Professional Association for Anthroposophic Art Therapy in Germany that took the initiative to start this work, in co-operation with the Medical Section and the Fine Arts Section at the Goetheanum.

Experts from the fields of sculpture, therapeutic drawing and painting, singing and instrumental music, and therapeutic speech came together to lay the foundation for a medical understanding of Man in artistic therapy. They started from basic questions such as: How can health and illness, as dynamic processes, be represented artistically? In what way is the work of art created by an artist different from the artistic process in the context of a therapy? How and where does art lead into the specifically therapeutic? How can the artistic understanding of Man, as developed by Rudolf Steiner in his fundamental lectures entitled *Art as seen in the Light of Mystery Wisdom*, be used to help us understand the healing effect of art? How can we investigate the concrete relationships between sound, form, colour and the specific activities of the organs of the human organism?

In view of the great variety of methodological approaches, and the broad spectrum of indications and therapeutic experiences of the therapists involved in the study groups, our intention was to single out the most relevant approach. We would also show the present state of anthroposophic art therapy in terms of today's available knowledge, understanding of illnesses and therapeutic application.

Since the overview we give needs to be short, the anthroposophical terminology we use can often only be introduced briefly. However, anybody interested can easily deepen their understanding with the help of the cross-reference and the bibliographical reference given at the back. A specific problem will arise with regard to the speech exercises which may easily sound simplistic, meaningless and incomprehensible to those not familiar with speech formation. However, we hope that just this will make some people interested in getting to know this form of artistic therapy by doing it themselves, which is easily possible in courses or individual sessions, even without any therapeutic intentions. To make the book more readable, we abstain from using the male and female grammatical form at the same time. Each should be thought of as being contained in the other.

The authors hope that this documentation will offer a representative overview of the way anthroposophic art therapy works at present, not only to doctors and therapists but also to a wider circle of people interested in the matter.

Introduction

Speech is an enormous continuous challenge towards higher and higher development.

Speech is our spiritual countenance which, like a traveller, we never cease to carry deeper and deeper into the unpredictable and unthinkable countryside of God.

Christian Morgenstern

The fact that voice training and speech training also contribute to man's wellbeing and health was shown already by the Hippocratic medicine and the Greek philosophers from the fourth century BC. This schooling of speaking was complemented by a number of gymnastic exercises, such as walking, running, jumping, wrestling, throwing the discus and the javelin as well as horse-riding. It was well known that physical exercise makes people more skilful in pronouncing the vowels and consonants and improves their ability to express themselves through speech. On the other hand, in those days, people still had deep respect for the word. The word did not merely serve the purpose of passing on information but was experienced as a powerful expression of the essence of the personality speaking — to the extent that words had a magic effect in the sense of curse and blessing, with the corresponding consequences for the people concerned.

In the second century AD natural-scientific research of anatomy and the physiology of the larynx started with Galen. Based on extensive vivisections of pigs Galen also described the functions of the innervation of larynx and speech apparatus.[1] During the Renaissance, it was Leonardo de Vinci who, with his numerous drawings of the larynx, fundamentally increased man's knowledge of the fine structure and the function of the speech instrument. He investigated the connection between speaking and breathing as well as the sound quality of words, giving an exact anatomical-physiological analysis of the functions of lips, tongue, velum, larynx and trachea as well as the nasal sinuses.

After the laryngoscope was developed by the English doctor Benjamin Guy Babington in 1829, the investigation of the neurophysiological and muscular processes of the functions of the larynx further progressed. Numerous works on the physiology of the human voice and on the Theory of Speech and its instruments were published. In the nineteenth century, clinical phoniatrics developed as the teaching of the anatomical-physiological foundations of voice and speech therapy in the form of a branch of

Introduction

Speech is an enormous continuous challenge towards higher and higher development.

Speech is our spiritual countenance which, like a traveller, we never cease to carry deeper and deeper into the unpredictable and unthinkable countryside of God.

Christian Morgenstern

The fact that voice training and speech training also contribute to man's wellbeing and health was shown already by the Hippocratic medicine and the Greek philosophers from the fourth century BC. This schooling of speaking was complemented by a number of gymnastic exercises, such as walking, running, jumping, wrestling, throwing the discus and the javelin as well as horse-riding. It was well known that physical exercise makes people more skilful in pronouncing the vowels and consonants and improves their ability to express themselves through speech. On the other hand, in those days, people still had deep respect for the word. The word did not merely serve the purpose of passing on information but was experienced as a powerful expression of the essence of the personality speaking — to the extent that words had a magic effect in the sense of curse and blessing, with the corresponding consequences for the people concerned.

In the second century AD natural-scientific research of anatomy and the physiology of the larynx started with Galen. Based on extensive vivisections of pigs Galen also described the functions of the innervation of larynx and speech apparatus.[1] During the Renaissance, it was Leonardo de Vinci who, with his numerous drawings of the larynx, fundamentally increased man's knowledge of the fine structure and the function of the speech instrument. He investigated the connection between speaking and breathing as well as the sound quality of words, giving an exact anatomical-physiological analysis of the functions of lips, tongue, velum, larynx and trachea as well as the nasal sinuses.

After the laryngoscope was developed by the English doctor Benjamin Guy Babington in 1829, the investigation of the neurophysiological and muscular processes of the functions of the larynx further progressed. Numerous works on the physiology of the human voice and on the Theory of Speech and its instruments were published. In the nineteenth century, clinical phoniatrics developed as the teaching of the anatomical-physiological foundations of voice and speech therapy in the form of a branch of the medical science. At the same time this also served to draw a clear line to logopaedia, introduced into speech therapy in 1924 by Fröschels as an independent discipline in the context of auxiliary healing professions.

Anthroposophical Therapeutic Speech adds a new integrative approach to healing speech education — logopaedia — and to the medical treatment of language and speech disorders — phoniatrics. By means of speech this therapeutic approach activates and exercises the spiritual, emotional and physical possibilities of movement and expression of the human being. This means that the act of speaking is seen in its relation to the whole anatomy and physiology of the body, not just in relation to the physiology of the larynx and the speech instrument in the narrower sense. For this reason Anthroposophical Therapeutic Speech is indicated not just for speech and language disorders, but also for a broad spectrum of physical and psychological diseases.

Speech not only expresses thoughts or encourages or discourages activities; on a very broad scale it also expresses the human world of emotions. This is shown not least by the great variety of philosophic-scientific, lyric and dramatic literature. Thus, consciously working on one's speech has an ordering effect on one's thinking, feeling and willing. This may prove particularly helpful in psychotherapy, after physical and emotional traumas, in the rehabilitation of drug addicts as well as the reintegration of juvenile delinquents.

Recent psycho-neuroimmunological research has shown to what extent the immune system depends on the psychological motivation as well as the inner strength and coherence of the personality in order to maintain health. It is this very coherence which is directly stimulated by the use of Therapeutic Speech. There is no other physical-psychological function through which we can express ourselves as individually and as personally as through our very individual way of speaking.

May this book contribute not only to describing the extensive therapeutic possibilities of speech, but also to rediscovering speaking and speech itself; that is to say, man's unique possibility to express himself and his relationship with the world and other people, and to work creatively with and on his speech. This will create a new possibility of self-development by means of artistic speech. A perspective of fundamental change will open up, as well as a new dimension of listening to and understanding the world around us. This new dimension, as a new quality of healing processes, needs to be developed and investigated.

Dr Michaela Glöckler
Medical Section, Goetheanum

PART ONE

Foundations of Therapeutic Speech

CHAPTER 1

Historical Development

Speech formation, or Creative Speech, is based on the ancient art of recitation and drama, revived and fundamentally redeveloped by Rudolf Steiner and Marie Steiner-von Sivers out of anthroposophy at the beginning of the twentieth century. It has had a stimulating effect on different areas, such as the arts, education, drama and therapy.[2]

The therapeutic work is based on the speech exercises given by Rudolf Steiner and on his numerous indications how to use the elements of speech therapeutically. This will be further expounded in the following chapters. All of Rudolf Steiner's speech exercises, developed in the years 1919 to 1924, were given to improve incorrect/imperfect speech, and most of them come with a clear medical indication. In this sense, the use of the whole range of more than sixty speech exercises is based on a diagnosis and is therefore therapeutic. Moreover, important therapeutic speech exercises were given for specific illnesses in other areas than the speech organism.

1.1 From the Beginning to the Present

In a hospital context, speech formation was first applied therapeutically between 1930 and 1936 in the former *Klinisch-Therapeutisches Institut* (now Ita Wegman Klinik) in Arlesheim, Switzerland, by Martha Hemsoth (January 29, 1887 – March 31, 1936) in cooperation with Dr Ita Wegman.

Martha Hemsoth and Ita Wegman first met at the end of the twenties. Martha Hemsoth was an opera singer by profession and probably decided in 1927 to do a training in speech formation. She finished her training with a diploma at the beginning of the thirties and started to work at the *Ita Wegman Klinik* soon afterwards. She worked with many patients but with doctors as well; moreover, she was in charge of arranging festivities artistically. Unfortunately, we know very little about her actual therapeutic work. In March 1936 she had an accident where she was seriously burned and died shortly afterwards. This fateful accident put an end to therapeutic speech work in the clinic for a long time.

Looking back over the last few decades, it has become obvious that therapeutic speech has thrived and developed wherever there has been a successful cooperation of one or more doctors with a therapist.

The further development of therapeutic speech in the area of somatic and mental illness in particular depends completely on this kind of cooperation. In the areas of education and curative education, where the need for speech therapy is much more obvious, anthroposophic therapeutic speech was able to unfold more easily within the various institutions.

1.2 Further Training

Nowadays, further training for doctors in principles of Therapeutic Speech takes place in Germany, Holland, Britain and Switzerland.

In Britain and Ireland, working groups of Therapeutic Speech Practitioners are regionally based. These groups are located in England (Southeast, West Midlands, Southwest), Scotland, Northern Ireland and Eire. The Anthroposophical Therapeutic Speech Association of Great Britain and Ireland (ATSA) is the professional association for practitioners and is the central point for the various regions. It organizes further training workshops and conferences and appoints mentors to oversee the training of new practitioners who take part in the In-Service Training Program. It is also the focal point for collecting case documentation, sharing resources and general professional support for association members. Plans are currently under way to develop a training that satisfies the standards set by Anthroposophical Health Professions Council.

1.3 Professional Associations

In Germany and Switzerland it is the responsibility of the respective Association for Anthroposophic Artistic Therapy (BVAKT and SVAKT) to represent the therapies to the outside world. These associations include all four of the Anthroposophic Art Therapies, namely painting, sculpting, music and speech formation, which are part of the anthroposophic doctor's therapeutic instruments.

In Great Britain the Therapeutic Speech Practitioner is registered with the Anthroposophical Health Professions Council (AHPC) and is a member of the Anthroposophical Therapeutic Speech Association of Great

Britain and Ireland (ATSA). Both the AHPC and ATSA represent Therapeutic Speech to the public. The AHPC is the registering body for all professionals in Anthroposophical Health Care and is concerned with profession standards and regulations.

1.4 Research and Recognition

As already mentioned in the introduction, it was in 1988 that the initiative for joint research was started to lay a systematic foundation for the Anthroposophic Art Therapies. For the next ten years different groups of doctors and therapists worked together for this purpose.

The 'Therapeutic Speech' group looked at the path of development speech took from art into education and then into medicine. As is well known, even the first speech exercises were developed in the context of the Waldorf School. Just as the child develops in natural stages, so different styles of poetry may be connected with individual age groups, where they are of particular benefit. Further subjects were:

— the speech elements of sound, voice, breath, vocalization, consonant formation
— the individual arts within speech
— the effectiveness of speech and the five types of disease; speech in connection with the bodily members
— rhythmic speaking

This book is the result of these meetings. Apart from recording individual case studies, systematic research was begun in various areas. Thus a study on the effect of therapeutic speech on the variability of the heart rate was drawn up, as well as a study on asthma patients. These projects were presented at a conference in the *Gemeinschaftskrankenhaus Herdecke* in 1998, where the further need for research was discussed as well.[3]

Today Therapeutic Speech, as a therapeutic method of anthroposophic medicine, is recognized and paid for by various health insurance companies in Switzerland, provided there is a supplementary insurance for complementary medicine. In Germany various health insurance companies will reimburse therapies prescribed by a doctor (some companies will review each case). In Britain Therapeutic Speech is privately funded by the patient. Some medical clinics offer bursary funding to offset therapy costs. Our aim is to have our profession recognized (after the appropriate training) as a medical auxiliary profession.

of inner intentions of the soul or the spirit. In the chapter 'The Breathing Human Being' we will go further into the significance of the air processes.

— **Air** brings about **lightness**
— **Air** causes **movement** which leads to **transformation.**
— **Air** conducts **light and warmth**, which brings about **brightening** and **enlivening**.

CHAPTER 3

Speech as Formed Exhalation

Speaking is the forming of the exhaled breath. With every consonant the stream of exhaled air is formed in a certain way and given corresponding tone vibrations by the vowels. Speaking always has an immediate effect on the breath; and any change of the exhalation has corresponding consequences for the inhalation. Working on the exhalation through which the word is created is an artistic process — the artistic means consisting of the various sounds, while the material that is being transformed is the air.

Speaking about speech we may quite naturally resort to a terminology that is connected to art. Speech may be called malleable or sculptured when the breath stream is shaped and formed by many strong consonants. When the sounds create the mood or the pictures, it is painting with sound. The music in language is experienced in the resounding vowels and in its inherent melody.

Above all, however, the process of speaking as such may be regarded as the archetype of any creative activity. When uttering a word the speech organs imprint the content of thinking into corresponding sound forms. In speaking the human being recreates the world of ideas in the stream of the outbreath. Thus his soul is provided with a means of expression.

This is the process of any creative activity: The idea (thought) is imprinted into the material (air) with the help of the appropriate instruments (tongue, teeth, lips). The material in turn changes. With regard to speech it is the element of air that is transformed into the carrier of sound and form.

Whoever speaks is living in a constant creative act, recreating in his exhalation the forms of the world in speaking. Be it the shapes of the outer world — tree, flower, stone or star; be it the soul's emotions or be it thoughts that he expresses in language: a person is always being creative and fully and entirely involved when bringing forth 'the word'. The finely coordinated motor activity of his speech instrument forms the sounds. With the help of his consciousness he comprehends the content of his speech, and the soul experiences what is being spoken, bringing the different nuances of tone and sound to his voice.

If the person speaking is in a situation where they struggle to find the appropriate words, the speaking process, which is otherwise unconscious and habitual, suddenly becomes comprehensible in its full creative potential. Likewise, somebody who cannot or is not allowed to express himself in words can feel his whole being stifled. It is as if violence is being done to the soul when the impulse to speak cannot express itself as word in the breath. One is '*condemned* to silence.' The idiom 'shut up' also expresses this.

Irrespective of whether someone has a connection to art, the very ability to utter words is a creative reality within them. If the human being actively takes hold of this potential, permeating the speech instrument with awareness and sensation, he finds himself immersed in a stream of living natural realities which make it possible for an *art* of speaking to emerge from the elements of everyday speech. Just as a sculptor transforms a natural rock into an artistically shaped sculpture by purposefully applying hammer and chisel in order to 'release the form hidden in the rock' (*Michelangelo*), so the speaker works on his natural speech and his ordinary habits of speaking and breathing, thus liberating and strengthening his personality that is caught in one-sidedness and often torn by contradictions.

By consciously taking hold of and working on his speech that is intimately connected with his whole being, the human being forms his exhalation and thereby forms himself right down into his physical body. In doing so creative forces are released on a larger scale.

CHAPTER 4

Artistic Means

The sounds of speech are the smallest unit in artistic speech and on these the therapeutic effect must be based. We need to distinguish between the sculpting consonants and the mood creating vowels. While the consonants give physical resistance to the stream of the breath and the voice by a stronger or softer use of the muscles, thereby exerting a formative influence on the air, the vowels simply reduce or extend the sound cavities giving the voice a certain coloration. These two groups of sounds — one produced by the activity of the various speech muscles, the other having its origin in the mood of the soul — are to be characterized below.

4.1 The Consonants

What is clearly audible, and can also be felt in the articulation process itself, is the reference of the consonants to the outer world. The consonants may be divided into four groups: impact sounds, wave sound, vibrating sound and blown sounds.[4] The four elements of earth, water, air and fire, which come to expression as solid, liquid, gaseous and warmth, are echoed in these groups.

In the tensing of the tongue and lip muscles the solidity of the impact sounds B, P, D, T and G, K may be experienced. The nasal sounds N and M bring a vibrating sensation to their basic impact quality. What is imitated in this group of sounds is the world of objects, of forms. In words like **b**all, **b**ear, **b**ead it is the round shape that is created and experienced, while in a**x**e, a**ct**ion and to **d**o it is the pure solid impact.

The wave sound L creates flowing movements, with the tongue very sensitively feeling the flow of the breath.

The air or vibrating sound R, on the other hand, can only be produced if uvula, tip of the tongue or lips allow themselves to *be moved* by the breath stream. The sound R gives itself completely to the element of air, particularly when it is a 'rolled' or trilled R. It is at home in the rolling and roaring of a river.

we think, feel and do becomes speech. If the intensity pressing outward in the /**u**/ is released a little, then with the help of the ring muscles of the lips the /**o**/ is formed — fuller and less dark in tone colour than the /**u**/. Delicately feeling back and forth between the two rear and the two front vowels the /**i**/ is formed behind the front teeth. The solidity of the teeth gives a radiating, directed quality to this vowel. Just as the /**o**/ begins to lighten up the darkness of the /**u**/, the /**e**/ mutes the brightness of the /**i**/ and consolidates itself deeper within the human being. In both the /**e**/ and the /**i**/ the voice stream is narrowed by the tongue as it is guided over the palate, while in the /**o**/ and /**u**/ it is the lips that narrow the resonance chamber.

The /**a**/ is the vowel that has the whole vault of the palate as a sound dome at its disposal, which is why in singing young children instinctively like to use it when carrying a melody (lalala.....). In the /**a**/ the soul experiences the world in amazement without restrictions and limitations. The stage curtain opens up: Ah! The sun rises: Ah!

With exclamations etc. where the soul moods are translated most directly and without hesitation into sound sensations, it is significant that people of joint language groups, no matter what age or social standing, use similar expressions:

a (as in /father/) — amazement about the world

e (as in /take/) — to become conscious of oneself (e.g. when speaking falters)

i (as in /free/)- to become strong in oneself (Also in defence.)

o (as in /fold/) — astonishment

u (as in /true/) — fear

aU (as in /down/) — pain (amazement immediately followed by contraction in fear)

aI (as in /high/) — tenderness

This means that, in the vowels, there is a kind of original language that everybody is familiar with, corresponding to the widening and contracting of the sound spaces. Changing the vowel while leaving the consonant unaltered, one can become aware when listening to the sound how it is not just the concept that changes but the fundamental mood of the soul as well: rum, rim, roam, room; sun, sane, sin, soon.

Looking at a word as a unity of vowel and consonant in the sense of the sound phenomena as described above, one may experience the following:

B — there is something solid. **LL** — Something round gets into a flowing movement. /**a**/ — the soul follows this in astonishment: **BALL**. Or /**o**/ — the soul lives into this in astonishment and love: **BOWL**.

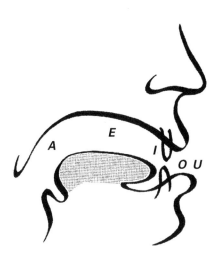

Figure 2: The positioning of the voice as it vocalizes.

4.3 Sound – Syllable – Word – Sentence – Gesture

The syllable is composed of consonants which recreate the outer world and vowels which characterize the world of the soul. In it outer and inner world unite to form a new, indivisible unity. The syllable is the image of archetypal language and as such the carrier of a spiritual wholeness.[7] The syllable is the first step into the creation of a word. Following the syllable step by step the human being masters a path through speech.

As soon as a syllable, or several syllables together, carry meaning, we are no longer dealing with a purely artistic phenomenon because thinking becomes involved in the newly created word. In the building of a word the syllable acquires rhythmic quality due to the stress pattern created. Moving from word to word, sentence dynamic arises which becomes most obvious in types of sentences, such as statement, imperative or question. A sentence can only be fully grasped and shaped if its gesture is comprehended. In everyday speaking, both for the speaker and the listener, these artistic elements of form and sound in speech retreat completely behind the information, the thought that is to be conveyed.

Only in poetry we do find the contents expressed according to the artistic laws of language, where speech is shaped through the means of sound imitation (onomatopoeia), rhythm, rhyme, stanza and the different stylistic elements such as the epic, lyric and dramatic styles.

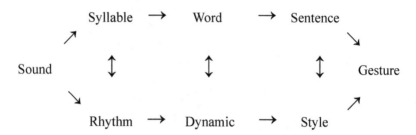

CHAPTER 5

Relationship Between the
Artistic Means and the Human Being

You must, when contemplating Nature,
Regard the whole, as well as every single feature:
There's naught within, there's naught without,
For what's within can be found without.
Therefore grasp with no delay
The sacred mystery, yet clear as day.
Take joy in true appearances,
Take joy in serious play.
No living thing is just one way,
But a multitude of many.

Johann Wolfgang von Goethe
(Trans. S. Eichstaedt)

The phenomena described in the preceding chapter are directly related to the human being. It is possible to draw certain conclusions about somebody's emotional and physical well-being according to the articulation region mainly used, how they intone their voice and how deeply their breathing is affected by their way of speaking. This is also where it is possible to exert an immediate therapeutic effect by changing the person's habits of speaking and breathing. For what the human being shapes with sound in the air works back physiologically on the organism.[8]

5.1 The Human Being and the Consonants

How the formative element of the consonants gives shape and clarity to our speech has already been described.[9] The better a person is mentally present in their words, the clearer their articulation will be. If somebody speaks out of emotions, rather, or if their consciousness is dull due to illness or exhaustion, their consonants will become weaker and their speech makes a difference whether the vowel is really experienced by the soul or whether, for instance, the latter refuses to open to the darkness of the /**u**/. In the /**a**/, forces of surrendering and letting go come to expression, in the /**e**/ the ability to consolidate oneself is expressed, while in the /**i**/ one asserts oneself. The /**o**/ contains mediating forces, and in the /**u**/ there lives the will to go through something with one's whole being. Since nowadays 80% of all diseases are of psychosomatic origin, these vocalic sound gestures may help to clarify many questions.[16]

The full, dark vowels /**a**/, /**o**/ and /**u**/ have a reference to the feeling and the will. The light and more pointed vowels /**e**/ and /**i**/, on the other hand, which are formed in the dental area, are related to the nervous system.

This, too, is audible in ordinary speech: While in the nervous person /**e**/ and /**i**/ are prevalent, which may easily give something shrill to the voice, the calmer, perhaps somewhat sluggish person colours his voice in the darker vowels /**a**/, /**o**/ and /**u**/.

The more the stream of the voice pushes towards the lips as in the /**u**/, the more intensity is needed; that is to say, the more demand is made both on the breath and the circulation. Following the sequence of the vowels /**a**/, /**e**/, /**i**/, /**o**/, /**u**/, the voice, and within it the soul, strives outward to the world. Conversely, in the sequence /**u**/, /**o**/, /**i**/, /**e**/, /**a**/, the soul opens up to receive the world.

In its wideness, /**a**/ is the most consonantal of the vowels, the one most closely related to the world, while the contracting quality of the sound /**u**/ makes the soul experience itself the strongest.[17]

— **Dark vowels: a, o, u, (aU)**
  Connected to the feeling and the will pole (blood vowels).
  A = opening up: giving oneself to the world
  U = Narrowing: strengthening one's personality

— **Light vowels: e, i, (aI)**
  Connected to the nerve-sense pole (nerve vowels).

5.3 The Breathing Human Being

The air processes, which through independent breathing become internalized, work on the human organism according to the same laws as the phenomena of the external air, as described above. Inert and heavy matter is brought into motion, into a circulation of transformation. Thus, the buoyancy of the red blood corpuscles, for instance, conveys the experience of lightness. Not only is free outer movement the result of this air process, but also cell metabolism, internal distribution of substances as well as the movement of the inner organs.[18]

The more regular and deeper the breathing is, the more life-filled and active the metabolic processes prove to be. The increased circulation and the warming of the body that goes along with it, is experienced by the human being quite consciously as enlivening and stimulating, both mentally and emotionally.

The human being may experience greatest freedom from the confinement and heaviness of the body when he imprints his thoughts, feelings and intentions of will into the stream of the outbreath, articulated in speech, thus imparting them to the external air and thereby to the world. There is no need even to leave the place where one is standing in order to reach the awareness, the heart of another person — who may be quite far away — with the air-borne words.

Each part of the human being is present in the exhaled air as carbon dioxide, moisture, movement and warmth. If speech is entrusted to the breath, it is moreover permeated with the force of thinking and the light of consciousness.

Since speaking always involves the breathing, any change of the breathing process has not only physical but also mental consequences. In healthy speaking, the inhaled breath is determined by what is to be spoken on the exhaled breath, with the soul quality playing a major role. One breathes in differently for a short exclamatory word than for a long sentence that is slowly unravelled. This is why influencing the breathing by means of a conscious speech formation has a deep-reaching effect.

All of the artistic means used in creative speech, such as sound, syllable, word, sentence, rhythm, dynamic, style or gesture, change the breathing when used consciously, influencing the latter's effect on body and soul in specific ways.

In classical Greek the word pneuma meant both the breath and the soul/spirit (also: *spiritus, ruoch, prana).*[19] In the Old Testament it is the divine breath that gives life and soul to the human body. In the rhythm of inhalation and exhalation a process can be sensed of the soul uniting with the body (incarnating) and then detaching itself again (excarnating), as also in waking and sleeping and, on a larger scale, birth and death.

As in the development of the child, the gradual deepening of the breathing goes together with the soul entering ever more deeply into the body. In the course of a life the physical organization is so thoroughly breathed through that soul qualities are actually released from the body, meaning a return to their spiritual origins.

With the help of the forces of inhalation the individuality takes hold of his body, warming it through and making it his own.[20] With the help of the forces of exhalation he turns back to the world, making use of the body in thinking, speaking and acting. If the individuality enters too deeply into the physical body, the latter becomes solid and hardened, turning from a meaningful tool of the ego into a kind of prison. In this way the mental soul processes as well as the organic processes are inhibited. If, on the other hand, the connection is too loose, the result is a lack of formative forces, uncontrolled organic processes and a certain desire to flee the earth.

The way somebody stands and walks is also the way they speak and breathe. The posture shows to what extent the human being has really taken hold of the forces of uprightness. Do they give in to gravity with a tendency to hardening, or do they tend to move in a way which suggests a certain desire to flee the earth? The knees should be observed as to how they hold the delicate equilibrium between gravity and lightness, and how this might relate to certain breathing habits.

The way people step also gives quite a differentiated picture of the movement sequences decisive for speaking and breathing. The therapist should study very carefully whether the way in which the foot is lifted off the ground is incited by an inner buoyancy, which would correspond to a healthy inhalation, or whether the feet shuffle along hardly leaving the ground. How do they reconnect with the ground: tentatively, heavily, in a stilted or skipping way or with a certain suppleness courageously feeling the ground? These observations can then be translated into a speech and breathing diagnosis.[21]

— **The Breath in the Organism:**
  Movement, buoyancy, combustion processes, transformation of substance.
— **Inhalation**: *Receiving of ego (incarnation, waking).*
— **Exhalation**: *Unfolding of ego (excarnation, sleeping).*

CHAPTER 6

'Knowledge of the Human Being' with Regard to Speech

In order to understand the approach of Therapeutic Speech it is necessary to know about certain results of spiritual scientific research which Rudolf Steiner developed into an anthroposophical knowledge of the human being, first with regard to education and then to medicine. The fundamental idea behind this image of man corresponds with what is said in the prologue of the St Johns Gospel where the whole world evolution is described as proceeding from the Word. However, of all creation the speaking human being alone has the ability to make free use of those forces from which he originates. He thus shares in a deeply creative process, recreating the creation of the world, as well as creating anew, changing and transforming, the world and himself. Thus the process of creation continues in himself and through himself, and in this way every therapeutic process is an example.

Within the human being himself certain systems work together and these appear mirrored also in the speech processes, as the following will show.

6.1 The Threefold Human Being

The human being lives in the polarity of mind and matter: he is a soul/spirit being in a living physical body. This polarity may also be called consciousness and life. Physically this is seen in the nerves and blood, or the nerve-sense system, on the one hand, and in the metabolic-limb system, on the other (see also Chapter 9 on Neurasthenia and Hysteria). In between the two we find the processes of the rhythmic system, stimulated by the heart and lungs, which have a mediating, harmonizing function between the upper and the lower systems.[22]

The breath combines articulation and voice, the representatives of nerve and blood in the speech, to a new wholeness: the syllable and the word.

The word, as it is being brought to birth, is embedded in the rhythm of in- and exhalation, and also works back upon this rhythm. The breath, transformed by the speech, strengthens and releases the voice, which in turn affects the blood organism.

Freeing the voice, and thereby strengthening the individual personality, is the prime task of any therapeutic speech treatment. A voice bound to the body, often experienced as pressure in and around the larynx, is an essential indication of a weakening in the whole organism.

As in the polishing of a precious stone, the voice is worked on by the speech instrument, cleaned and polished by the consonants, so that, purified and healed, it may unfold to reveal its deepest beauty.[26]

— **Head**
  Thinking
  Nerve-sense organization

— **Lungs/heart**
  Feeling
  Rhythmic system

— **Arms/ legs/ stomach**
  Willing
  Metabolic-limb system

6.2 The Bodily Members and their Involvement in the Speech Process

Just as the voice (the vowel element) bears witness to the feeling of well-being in the thinking, feeling and willing human being, revealing the way in which he is incarnated, so the formation of the consonants is echoed in and supported by the fourfold physical organization, the resistance of which awakens the consciousness for speech. This fourfoldness is based on the four bodily members of the human being. They are the basis of the anthroposophical knowledge of man and of anthroposophical medicine.[27]

In the human being four levels of being and of consciousness are differentiated, the outer expression of which is the solid physical body, the balance of fluids, the breathing organism and warmth. Each of them corresponds to and lives in association with one of the four realms of nature: mineral, plant, animal and human being.

The mineral, **the stone**, shows itself to be solid matter which cannot change of its own accord. It consists only of a **physical body** and is subject to the laws of matter.

The plant, with its ability to grow, assimilate and propagate itself, is alive. Only when it dies, that is to say when the life force withdraws, does it disintegrate into its material components. This means that it does not only have a physical-material body but also a **life or ether body**.

The animal, on the other hand, is able to move about freely according to its drives and instincts, unlike the stone and the plant. With the help of sounds and particular behaviour patterns it is able to express increasing variations of soul moods the higher it is developed. In addition to the physical and the ether body, the animal has a **soul body**, or **astral body**.

In the **human being** we distinguish the physical body which, left to itself after death, is without consciousness and completely subject to the laws of lifeless matter. It is permeated by the life or ether body to which a kind of sleeping consciousness is attributed. Thus, in a sleeping or comatose person the life processes will continue unhindered for a time, similar to the life processes in plants.

When awake, the human being's physical and etheric structure is permeated with the soul or astral body which gives him a dreaming consciousness, similar to all creatures. However, only the human being has an **ego** or **I**, and is therefore aware of himself. It is the ego that allows him to control himself, to change himself, to be a unique individual.

These four bodily members correspond to the four elements of earth, water, air and fire which, as described before, are reflected in the four groups of consonants.[28]

Earth:	**Physical body**	*(impact sounds: D, T, B, P, G, K, M, N)*
Water:	**Life body or ether body**	*(wave sound: L)*
Air:	**Soul body or astral body**	*(air sound or vibrating sound: R)*
Fire:	**Ego or I**	*(warmth/blown sounds: H, CH, J, SH, S, F, W)*

There is also a connection between the three placement zones and the four members mentioned above, with the physical body constituting the basis for speaking. The sensitive but distinct borderline of the lips is connected to the **ego**. In the sharpness and alertness of the teeth placement the liveliness of the **astral body** makes itself felt. The more unconscious region of the rear palate dome, which is closer to the life processes, reveals a connection to the **ether body** and its formative forces. Working on the individual placements has a stimulating and strengthening effect on the corresponding members. Thus, for instance, withdrawing or setting boundaries is a faculty of the ego organization. A person unable to control their bladder, usually shows also weakness and lack of muscle control in the lips. Thus working on the lip sounds, the impact sounds in particular, has a strengthening and balancing effect.

Lip sounds:	**Ego**	Feeling
Tongue/teeth sounds:	**Astral body**	Thinking
Palate sounds:	**Ether body**	Will

What is truly human can be experienced only when the ego activity is not limited to itself but begins to work on the other members which, consequently, undergo a transformation. The human being then begins, to a certain degree, to become independent of drives and passions or the needs of the body.

With time a transforming of the soul/astral body allows a new quality to arise: the **Spirit-self.** Unlike the astral body not yet transformed by the Powers of ego, the Spirit-self, purified from desires, becomes the bearer of the spirit.

The ability also to transform ether and physical body with the help of the ego still needs to be developed in the distant future. Then, the life or ether body will be transformed into the **Life-spirit**, and the physical body into the **Spirit-man**. (See also later in this chapter 'Speech and its Relation to Other Arts'; and Chapter 13, 'Processes of Development'). This means that the human being has the possibility to transform the given four bodily members, creating his true sevenfold nature. In order to understand this process better, let us look at the archetypal plant as developed by Goethe: *seed (germ), leaf, bud, blossom, stamen, fruit, seed (grain).*

Plant

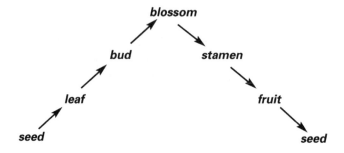

The following diagram shows the relationship between the human development and the plant. The ascending line on the left shows what is given by the Creator, the descending line on the right shows what is created by the ego.[29]

Human being

spiritual		*ego*	
ensouled	*astral body*	Spirit-self	
alive	*ether body*		Life-spirit
material	*physical body*		Spirit-man

The activity of these bodily members can be observed at different stages of the forming of language. The physical body alone can produce nothing but noises. It serves as a tool to bring about the sound formation inherent in the etheric body of the human being. The mother tongue, which the child adopts without understanding in a dream-like imitation, is a force forming his body and soul — a force that may also work habitually in sleep without any consciousness at all.

How very different, on the other hand, does speech sound when a variety of nuances of the soul become audible. The impulse to speak is in the *astral body*: It is always the soul that wants to express itself in the spoken word, seeking the conversation with the other soul.[30] The further developed the personality is, the more clearly the speech process may be directed by the ego. This makes it possible to become more independent of habitual speech patterns (e.g. a dialect or speech idiosyncrasies adopted from one's parents). Such a person will choose the right words for their thoughts and feelings, will be able to remain silent when necessary, while the kind of speech instigated mainly by the soul seeks spontaneous, often premature, expression — which is so charmingly seen in children.

Freeing oneself from the habitual in one's speech also makes it possible to learn foreign languages which, in turn, help us to become more independent of the habitual.

In a similar way we can almost relearn our own mother tongue with the help of speech formation by uniting with our speech through conscious activity and experiencing. In doing so the ego orientates itself by the laws of speech rather than by inclination and habit, which is a first step towards transformation of the bodily members. The speech impulse consciously seized by the ego always means a warming-through of the breath organism, which in itself supports the transformation of the astral body.

All speaking is possible precisely because the human being has an *ego*, sovereign over the other members of his being. Only an 'Ego among egos'

aware of how different the world sounds in various little poems and word games.

The different **styles of speech** are an expression of the fourth effect of speech. The differentiated way of forming the epic, lyric and dramatic placements, the declamatory or recitative way of speaking as well as the different poetic styles all have an *awakening* effect on the soul. This is an element the child should absorb up to Class 5. Around the age of eleven the child's breath has become deep enough to enter into a relationship with the blood system.

This brings about a new connection between body and soul. Gradually a constant pulse-breath quotient develops. (This process, which according to Rudolf Steiner is imperative for establishing the so-called 'maturity of the breath,' is helped by working with declamatory alliteration in Class 4, thereby deepening the breath. In Class 5, when blood and breath have started to communicate with each other, the children work in the recitative style of the very rhythmic hexameter, thus harmonizing the processes of body and soul.) [38]

The laws inherent in speech will finally lead the human being to the **gestures** underlying the words, thereby revealing their real nature. By working on the basic gestures of speech (see 8.4, **Additional Therapeutic Speech Elements**) the speaker as a whole is turned into an instrument of speech, thus undergoing a self-determined, *purifying* transformation of his own self. The speech gesture, which makes the fundamental gesture of beings and things *audible* in the musical-plastic formation of the word, transforms what is spatial into something temporal, and what is material into something living-etheric: it is of superior spiritual quality. (Around the age of fourteen the adolescent begins to dissociate himself from anything previously given, searching for himself as well as the sense and nature of the world. This inner drama and the necessary reorientation around the time of his 'earthly maturity' is prepared by means of poetic ballads. A theatre play around this age moreover offers the adolescent the opportunity to immerse himself into a new role, body and soul.)

The above-mentioned five effects of speech give an archetypal image of the healthy human being and harmonious development. Starting from the ego the physical body is seized and shaped by the sound formation. Rhythm is the foundation of anything living and is an expression of the nature of the etheric organization. The astral body, on the other hand, moves in differentiated, dynamic processes. The ego, awaking when confronted with a different style, is given an opportunity to understand itself and reveal its own spiritual nature.

The schooling path of speech formation (creative speech), as developed by Rudolf Steiner and Marie Steiner-von Sivers, is based on the above-mentioned laws of the knowledge of the speaking human being. They were put into words by Christa Slezak-Schindler who has worked with them for decades.[39]

In the first five exercises for articulation (*Dart may these boats… — Proxy prized*; see Chapter 8) they are already present in rudimentary form and further differentiated and evolved in subsequent exercises.

Clear Speaking	forms the organs
Rhythmic speaking	has an ordering effect
Dynamic speaking	frees and strengthens
Stylistic speaking	has an awakening effect
Gesture-filled speaking	has a purifying effect

6.4 Speech and its Relation to Other Arts[40]

The speech organism, and the human form which develops from it, represents an instrument created by the spirit of language: an instrument used and brought into movement by the ego. This point of view is an essential foundation of the anthroposophic knowledge of man, explained in many different ways.[41] This is the aim of human development: to become an individual personality (Latin: *personare* — to sound through).

The human being as a 'construction' is *speech architecture*. The latter determines in what way the human being is able to unfold in speaking. With the help of the speech organs *plastic sound forms* are produced in the air. Just as a potter works clay, a sculptor wood or stone, so the speech artist works the sound gestures into the outstreaming breath. *Soul colours* emerge when, in speaking, the breathing rhythm enfolds both the light of thinking and the unconscious will processes into a living wholeness in the consonantal-vocalic creation of the word. As soon as the rhythm of breathing and speaking come together, colourful pictures arise in the soul. With *prosody* (melody) and *intonation* the voice gives life to them: what is normally visible in space becomes audible in the stream of time, and by creating the sound the ego liberates itself.

Poetry, which gives poetic expression and use to speech, is based on the different elements of style. The poetic word works as far down as into the rhythmic life processes, when understood in its essence. The speech organism, too, is transformed in working on the different placements.

The *eurythmic gesture* lives invisibly in the artistically formed voice as sound form and soul gesture. Thus the elements of syllable step, sound form and gesture, appearing as movements of the physical body in eurythmy, are created in the listening space. The voice, and the blood organism it is based on, can more and more purify itself from egoism by letting themselves be transformed by the speech forces. This gives a notion of how, in the distant future, man will have permeated himself with speech to such an extent that his whole physical organization is transformed into a creative breathing process. This will be the Spirit man, the breathing aspect of man, transformed through the word.[42]

6.5 Therapeutic Speech and Eurythmy Therapy

Both therapeutic speech formation and curative eurythmy work with the healing forces of speech. Eurythmy is the sister of the art of speech: by using physical movements it makes *visible* what speech makes *audible*. This means that both forms of therapy have the same origin: Speech. However, while eurythmy works with the 'big man' of the metabolic-limb system, therapeutic speech formation works through the 'little man,' the archetypal image, of the speech organism.

Thus, eurythmy heals through the individual *sound* or *sound sequence* which adjusts the macrocosmic formative forces of the sound to the respective symptoms. Forming the sound in movement, those processes which have become one-sided are readjusted to a healthy balance.

The therapeutic speech practitioner and the patient are very directly confronted with the disease and its psychosomatic origins. This is the reason why therapeutic speech, for instance, works mainly with *whole words, syllables and sentences*, since the combination of sound and voice (consonant and vowel) in the word is something like a natural bridge between psyche and soma.

Working from the ego with the main expression of the astral body, i.e. speech, therapeutic speech is directly confronted with the cause of numerous diseases. Especially with somatic diseases this is often to be found on the different levels of the astral body, as has been confirmed by recent studies, for instance in psycho-oncology. This means that the effect of therapeutic speech starts at the very centre of the disease, from where it can spread out and broaden in an harmonizing way.

Eurythmy therapy, on the other hand, starts from the archetype of the sound in the metabolic-limb system of the human being, bringing the healing forces to the diseased organ.[43] For both forms of therapy, however, the premise is that the human body is formed by cosmic sound forces, the effect of which was described accurately by Rudolf Steiner. These sound forces may be localized in the body in detail and put to therapeutic use.

Observing these two healing arts it becomes obvious that in eurythmy, the artist or patient immerse themselves in the forces of the periphery with their limbs, letting those forces stream in — a process which takes place *invisibly* in speech with every inhalation. The audible beginning of formed speech lies in the formative force of the sounds, which is *centred* in the speech organs. Starting from that force, the speaker then extends into the periphery again via the outbreath.

Going through the metabolic-limb system eurythmy begins to take effect directly in the etheric from where it then works on the rest of the system. Therapeutic speech, on the other hand, starts in the rhythmic system and works on ego and etheric body, starting from the astral body.

Experience has shown that these two forms of anthroposophic therapy complement one another extremely well. Sometimes it is necessary for patients to do eurythmy therapy first, in order then to be able to experience speech in a new way. Likewise it can be a good preparation for those people who are not yet ready to confront their disease in so conscious a way. Those patients, however, wanting to approach their difficulties directly, may find it very satisfying to start with speech; often they can then truly connect with eurythmy at a later time.

CHAPTER 7

General Diagnosis in
Therapeutic Speech

In therapeutic speech the diagnosis is based on the five main criteria: stance — breathing — voice — articulation — and thinking. Most diagnoses, in all the different areas where therapeutic speech is applied, are made according to these criteria; however, they can be done in various ways. Numerous colleagues, for instance, use the five criteria on their own in an individual order. But it is just as well possible to structure each of the five areas in detail according to the four members, leading to a deeper understanding of the diseases and an intensive dialogue with anthroposophical doctors and other artistic therapists.

The following explanations are referring mainly to therapeutic speech with adults referred on the basis of psychiatric, psychosomatic and somatic indications. For speech disorders the respective aspect of this diagnosis will be further differentiated later in the book.[44]

The Diagnosis

The question now is how exactly this scheme can be helpful in making a diagnosis in each case. By doing basic exercises the therapist will attempt, in the course of the first sessions, to get a basic picture of the patient's speech and will become aware of certain characteristics. In the case of depression, for instance, these may refer to all five areas or, as in the case of functional dysphonia, may be limited mainly to the breath and the voice. These characteristics are then assigned to the corresponding bodily member(s) in the scheme leading to a limited number of affected areas (i.e. three to five). Based on this diagnosis appropriate steps in the therapeutic process can then be planned and the resulting changes be followed up. Since we are dealing here with an artistic therapy, these changes are to be described in qualitative terms. Thus, for instance, the connection between the vowels and the consonants may be disturbed at the level of *the astral body* in the area of the *voice*. Although the patient may be speaking the consonants well, their voice may be 'stuck in the throat' so that they cannot make the vowels resound clearly behind the teeth. This can be improved in the course of the therapy leading to a clear dental placement.

In practice, the simple form of diagnosis according to certain main characteristics in the five areas will normally be sufficient. In complicated cases, however, the patient's ability to express himself may be observed in each of the twenty fields, thus enabling the therapist to make a comprehensive diagnosis.

Deviation or Disease?

It is important to observe the difference between deviations from the ideal, which are still at the functional level, and proper diseases, even if this difference is often a subtle one. In many cases this differentiation will have to be made in cooperation with the doctor.

However, due to the close connection between the organism as a whole and the speech instrument, many diseases do manifest themselves directly in the patient's speech and may be considerably improved by working at the level of the speech.[45] Colitis, for instance, nearly always goes along with a distinct weakness of the labial sounds and certain vocal symptoms, even if no speech or voice disorder has been diagnosed.

In formulating a diagnosis and planning the course of therapy it must be distinguished whether a disease expresses itself clearly as a deviation in the five areas and is treated as such (e.g. asthma), or whether one is dealing with a primary disorder/disease in one of the five areas (e.g. functional dysphonia). In the latter case, an underlying problem may be inferred, such as a professional overstraining of the voice. The human being as a systemic whole will express all his conditions with seismographic accuracy in the central area of speech.

	STANCE	BREATHING	VOICE	ARTICULATION	THINKING
EGO	Uprightness, gait, state of warmth, shape of body, body language, way of thinking.	Orientation of breath; directing of breath. Way of dealing with sense impressions, 'light and soul breathing.' Depth of incarnation.	Identification with one's own voice. Pitch. 'Core' of the voice (individuality) Directing of the voice. Intonation.	Clarity and structure of speech. Grip (ego presence) in the four sound groups (consonants).	Power and span of concentration. Clarity of thoughts. Comprehension. Vocabulary. Richness. Sentence structure. Memory.
ASTRAL	Manifestation of thinking, feeling and willing. Relationship to the directions in space. Character; gestures; attitudes; muscle tone; flow of movement.	Ability to breathe in and out pleasure and pain (sentient body), joy and sorrow (sentient soul), or to 'freeze.' Focus on breathing in, on breathing out, in sympathy/antipathy. Impulse and strength of breathing. Influence on breathing rhythm. Day pulse breath quotient.	Strength and modulation of the voice. Connection between vowels and consonants. Ensouling (thinking, feeling, willing). Vocal quality. Sound quality. Vocalization. Six gestures.	Gripping of placements. Force of articulation. Speech impulse. Three places of articulation (thinking, feeling, willing) placement. Ability for word gesture. Sound quality of the vowels.	Interest. Cleverness. Thoughtfulness. Fluency of thoughts. (Imperative/long and winding sentences.)
ETHERIC	Constitution; buoyancy; lightness. Liquid conditions. Temperament. Turgor. Shape of the body.	Type of breathing (shallow, deep, mixed). Focus on breathing out. Breathing capacity. Breathing as a rhythmical life process. Breathing flexibility. Night pulse breath quotient.	General impression of the voice: family similarities, ethnic origin (heredity). Flexibility and flow, volume and constitution of the voice. Euphonia/dysphonia.	Speech habits in mother tongue, environment, dialect. Functional articulation disorders. Speech disorders. Strength to form sounds (sound gesture).	Matrix of memory: long-term memory, memory for music or language.
PHYSICAL	Physiological function of the body. Outer appearance: fat, thin; big-headed, small-headed (see ego). Condition of speech instruments.	Mouth/nasal breathing. Narrow or wide air cavities. Condition of respiratory organs.	Sounding spaces. Condition of larynx and diseases.	Morphological deviations. Condition of instrument. Dysarthria, dyspraxia.	Condition of brain. Soundness or disorder of sense organs. Cerebral disorders, injuries, tumors etc. Aphasia.

Table 2: Diagnosis

overcome the dominant forces of the hereditary body (meaning, in the extreme, physical or mental handicap)?[47]

Another breathing rhythm is the change between sleeping and waking up. This change, too, is of considerable interest to speech, since a person who sleeps too much needs to be treated differently from a person suffering from a lack of sleep. The question then is: are we dealing with a problem of going to sleep or waking up?

Another breathing process of the soul and the ego may be called '*light and soul breathing*'[48] This means the very subtle inhalation and exhalation through sense perceptions. With regard to the eyes this process may be explained in terms of seeing and looking. Seeing and grasping something may be compared to inhalation. Only when looking closely at something for a longer time is a response given by the soul and a feeling results. In this feeling, ego and soul can stream out again.

This ability to look finds expression in any good nature poetry. Nowadays most people rush from one impression to the next ('... I've already seen that...') and consequently are flooded by sense impressions: there is too much 'sensory inhalation.' As a consequence the ability of the upper organization to concentrate is weakened and the constitution is damaged (neurasthenia); it may even cause organic disease. As speech artists we have an essential therapeutic tool against such one-sidedness at our disposal — namely poetry. The soul's ability to inhale and exhale must be included into the diagnosis.

The way somebody breathes while speaking shows the ability of the ego to lead and direct the breath. Is the breath able to direct the person's speech into width, height and depth? Can the breath be matched with the length of the line?

Breathing and Astral Body

Rate, depth and dynamics of the breath are determined by astral and etheric body. Thus, the breath should always respond in a subtle way to emotional experiences, communicating them to the body. Any blockage or constriction will result in problems and/or disorders. How does the patient breathe when experiencing *joy or pain*? Can emotional experiences find their way into the speech via the breath?

Have negative experiences and a negative attitude to the world also made the breathing shallow and narrow? The breathing of a healthy child around the age of twelve can here serve as a model.

In people who do a lot of sports the breathing is often deep and regular, but only oriented even in waking towards the physical, lacking connection to the inner life.

By getting too involved in situations, the inability to set boundaries, and therefore a lack of independence, tends to over-emphasize the process of inhalation in the broadest sense and may predispose to cancer. The pulse breath quotient as well as the respiratory sinus arrhythmia also shows how the astral body takes hold of the breath.

A quotient above four at rest normally indicates that the person is breathing very slowly, which often results when the upper organization is strongly orientated towards the world and there is little healthy self-perception. This is a typical expression of our present civilization in the breath.

Breathing and Etheric Body

In this area we are concerned with the type of breathing, insofar as it is the expression of a chronic condition. Are we dealing with habitual *shallow, deep or 'mixed' breathing*? Is the breathing able to sustain its vital function properly? Here, spontaneous breathing and breathing while speaking have to be looked at separately. *Maximum volume and peak flow of the breath* will also say something about the condition of the etheric body and possible disturbances of its healthy rhythms. These may result, for instance, when astral body and ego activity exert an irregular influence on the other members (e.g. asthma).

The general question here is: Does the patient have a healthy *spontaneous breathing* when speaking? If not, which aspects of his breathing need to be improved?

The *flow of speech* is also based on the way the breath is directed. This is why fixated disfluencies (stuttering) fall into this area.

Breathing and Physical Body

The *constitutional* and *morphological* conditions of the lungs, the bronchi, the trachea, the larynx, the glottis, as well as the nose with its sinuses and the frontal sinus can affect the breathing. With adults these influences are often fixed and unchangeable. And yet it is often amazing to watch how strong and deep the breath may become despite these limiting conditions.

Important for the therapist is to check if the patient breathes through the mouth or the nose, both by day and by night, especially with children.

Further information about pathological changes in this area may also be obtained via an ENT diagnosis.

Voice and Ego

The voice is an expression of the personality. Often we can recognize a person by the sound of his voice, even before understanding words. What is of diagnostic interest is a person's relationship to his own voice.

The *pitch* tells us something about how deeply the person is incarnated in their body (soprano, alto etc.). However, one has to remember that due to a wrong use of the voice, as well as tensions, the speaking voice is often not at its natural pitch. Is a central *core* audible in the voice (ego presence)? Can the voice be directed? One has to take into consideration that practice plays a considerable part. Directing the voice is the ability to alter consciously modulation, dynamics etc.

Voice and Astral Body
The strength of the voice and its natural modulation are influenced by the astral body. On the whole, under this heading, the musicality of the voice is of interest. Since any emotion can express itself in the voice, working with the voice also means working with the soul and the personality. Thinking, feeling and willing each have a different influence on the voice which may limit its free unfolding, both by one-sided thought processes and dominant will forces.

The patient's ability or inability to *bring vowels and consonants together* gives important information about the way astral body and etheric body are connected. Can the vowel receive the formative force of the consonant (aim of the therapy) making the voice resound, or does the vowel remain separate? Does the vowel dominate the word?

Concerning the *onset of voicing*, the following distinctions can be made: breathy, gentle, firm and hard (pressed). These qualities give the therapist an idea of how the astral body takes hold of the voice.

On the whole, of particular interest is *the way the astral body deals with the vowels*. A preference for one or the other vowel suggests that the soul likes to dwell in the corresponding vowel gesture. The six qualities of speech (soul gestures) also find expression mainly through the vowel. This shows that it is possible to start from the voice in order to learn about soul qualities or else to look for an impression of corresponding moods in the voice. Decisive for the health of the voice is an harmonious connection between the soul (intention) and the available etheric-physical means of expression.

Voice and Etheric Body
Many qualities of the voice have their origin in the etheric body. They are influenced by hereditary forces such as family similarities as well as the specific way the voice sounds in a person's mother tongue. The tonal range of the voice (e.g. over two octaves) as well as the constitution of the voice also belong under this heading. Both may be changed to a certain extent by way of training the voice. In many people years of incorrect use of the voice have impaired the way the voice sounds, e.g. in hyperfunctional dysphonia. This is often found in professional speakers whose voice

problems are due to wrong speaking habits; in the beginning emotional strain passes into the speech (astral body) with the problem gradually slipping down into the etheric (as habit). This example shows that astral body and ether body are closely interconnected in the area of the voice.

Voice and Physical Body
Here the size and constitution of *larynx and resonance caves* are of interest. Years of incorrect use of the voice may cause vocal nodules, thus leaving an imprint in the physical body. Likewise, *diseases* leading to, for instance, paralysis of the vocal folds or tumors manifest themselves in this area. As already mentioned in connection with the breath, the decisive factor is the way the voice is used. This means that the most frequent origin of voice problems lies in the area of the astral or the etheric.

Articulation and Ego
Many aspects of articulation are influenced by the ego. This is shown clearly by the fact that any impairments have a negative effect on articulation. Such impairment may be due to tiredness, illness or exogenous factors, such as alcohol or drugs.

The qualities of articulation of interest here are the *clarity and structuring* of speech as well as the ability to shape the *four consonant groups* (breath, impact, vibrating and wave sounds).

A further faculty of the ego is to hold the balance between the different aspects of speech. Focusing on this balance will school the ego. A strong imbalance, irrespective of other characteristics, suggests a lack of ego presence in that person's speech. Articulation is determined most strongly by the ego.

Articulation and Astral Body
The three consonantal placements in particular relate to the astral body.[49] The labial sounds (M, B, P — F, V, W) are formed at the borderline between inside and outside and are connected to feeling. The sounds of the dental placement (L, N, D, T, S, Z — SH) are the result of the tongue acting in combination with the hardest substance in the body, the teeth. This contrast brings about awareness, and consequently the dental placement is connected with thinking. The velar sounds (G, K, H, Y, NG — and CH like in the Scottish 'loch') are formed furthest back in the speech instrument and are an expression of the will pole of speech.

Since each of these three placements is connected either with the heart and breast area, the brain and spinal cord or with the human form down to the heels, one may also infer a connection between weakness within individual placements and the area of stance.

Does a person have a preference for imperative sentences and a generally precise style, or does he place sub-clause next to sub-clause, like leaves on a stem? These elements of speech diagnosis are part of the characteristics of a person and largely not to be considered pathological.

Thinking and Etheric Body

Thoughts achieve their fundamental mood because at this level one's temperament is situated: fiery – idealistic; airy – intimate, many-sided; watery – imaginative; solidly – clear constructive and schematic.

The etheric body is the matrix for the memory. A rich life of thought can only develop on a firm basis of health. If health is present then thought can be expressed in the language. Conversely, the way of thinking will also have a forming influence on the etheric body. Is it kept fresh by an active thought life and assimilation of life experience? Is it constantly being renewed by a lively way of perceiving, by artistic activities? The memory (experiences imprinted into the etheric body) also belongs to this level. What is also of interest is that often there seems to be a difference between memory for speech and memory for music. Speech is remembered more by the limbs while music is remembered more by the head.[50]

Thinking and Physical Body

Both the expressive and the receptive assimilation of thoughts in speech is dependent on *the healthy functioning of certain parts of the brain*. Consequently a variety of disturbances of this assimilation are part of this area. Apoplexies, tumors, lesions etc. impairing the cerebral function will result in the different types of aphasias, such as motor, amnesic, semantic, or total aphasia.[51]

In general, when this level is affected there is a neurological diagnosis to take into consideration.

CHAPTER 8

Aspects of Therapy

8.1 Cause and Cure of Illness

The breath is the archetype of all mediating and transformative forces and forms the basis of all metabolic processes. Whether we process a mental thought, digest food material or 'breathe away' an emotional experience — in all of these instances we are dealing with a rhythmical breathing process in a broader sense. This can be seen as taking in, changing and giving out, as described above.

Whenever we take a breath in order to speak, it is not just air that we inhale but the inhalation is influenced by what we want to say, and subsequently filled with it. Here the rule applies that you cannot give out what you have not first taken in. Moreover, the inhalation will be different according to what the person is going to say and how they are going to say it. This means that the elements and laws of speech taken in upon inhalation are of therapeutic significance. What we have taken in will set the impulse; thus, speaking may be understood as a reaction to the impulse we have inhaled — a process easily comprehensible when compared with physical nourishment.

While the impulses inhaled are filled with formative, sculptural forces, the exhalation has a loosening and musical quality.

The turning point of inhalation and exhalation is the actual moment of ego activity which lifts the polarities of spirit and matter, consciousness and life (the equivalent of which is inhalation and exhalation) into an integrated rhythmic process. This process can be found in all parts of the human organism. Variations of the dialogue between inhalation and exhalation are expressed in the way nerves and blood interact. However, this dialogue also becomes visible in the division of the conscious and unconscious nervous systems, the venous and arterial blood circulation, and the activity of individual organs, while the glandular organization shows to what extent the life processes respond to impulses of mind and soul by way of excretion. Therefore, joy or pain, pleasure or frustration have a stimulating or stifling effect on the organism, showing as released or held breath.

It is the breath that builds the bridge from spirit and soul to the physical and etheric.

If the relationship between inhalation (what is taken in) and exhalation (what is given away) is disturbed or if there is congestion at the turning point between the two, the human being will become ill. The disorder may be of a psychic, a psychosomatic or an organic nature. Our health very much depends on whether the metabolic processes of body, soul and spirit are circulating in the right way and that this stream is not interrupted. The circulation is a 'continuous process of healing' which is sparked and ordered by the breath.

'In every instance of internal healing we need to help the breathing process, which continues into the body as a whole, in such a way that everywhere in the human being it may reconnect the process of circulation with the general conditions in the cosmos.'[52]

This is where speech as a therapy begins. When breathing conditions, which are largely disturbed today, reorient themselves towards speech and its laws, the circulation again experiences cosmic regulation, since the laws of speech correspond to cosmic world laws.

The sounds and rhythms in particular are administered to the sick breathing, like a remedy, by way of very specific exercises. Rudolf Steiner's statement that *'All secrets of healing are at the same time secrets of breathing'*[53] have been put to immediate practice in his work and exercises with speech and breath. The health and strength-giving effect of the breath depends on whether the astral body is able to open up and take in the ego; that is to say, on whether the soul is actively involved during inhalation or whether it has become fixed in the physical and thus blocks the inhalation.

If the soul opens up to speech joyfully and actively, the lungs will grow wider to receive the ego. Specific gestures may further increase this widening. The ego may then become active in the physical organization, warming it through and bringing about the necessary transformation of the substances taken into the body.

Following the syllable step and rhythm of speech into the air and listening to the tone as it is set free, the soul experiences a widening and loosening in the exhalation. By means of 'the art of breathing' which may be relearned in the process of speaking, 'man frees himself from those earthly influences that make him ill,'[54] and his whole being becomes brighter and lighter. Of particular significance in this context is the intake of iron which is increased by the kind of inhalation oriented towards spirit and soul, forming and strengthening the organism (*see case study on anaemia*).

A specific question to be asked by the therapist is in what way the breathing and circulation conditions of the diseased organs have been damaged; whether there is a balance between the forming and loosening elements, between lightness and gravitation, movement and rest, etc.

Increased activity of speaking and breathing supports the activity of the organs. Deeper blockages, such as shocks, traumas and even mineral deposits and stones may thus gradually be dissolved and 'breathed out.' The person prone to inflammatory diseases will receive the formative forces he needs via the breath.

The depressive will be able to reconnect with the forces of lightness in the inhalation. The asthmatic will learn to disentangle his exhalation from its nerve-sense connection, integrating it back into the life processes (see Chapter 10, '*Observations of Some Illnesses*').

The two speech disorders of **stuttering** and **lisping** are archetypes of overly hardened and overly loose incarnations. The breath of the stutterer gets stuck in the sound formation and runs up against it until he manages at last to release the stream of breath through the articulation. The lisping person is struggling with the problem of experiencing and respecting the body as a boundary giving hold and support. Breathing out he slips right through this boundary, as it were. From the point of view of speech one may say that while the stutterer dives too deeply into the bodily member-building forces of the articulation, the lisping person does it too little.

Typically it is the earth sounds (B, P, D, T, G, K) which make the stutterer experience the resistance of the body so strongly, while the lisping person strives to exit the body with the blown sounds.[55] The formation of every consonant may be looked at in terms of whether there is too much or too little formative force. What is important to note, therefore, is the group of sounds and the placement where the articulation is too strong or too weak.

The breath, more than any other medium, seems to be able to reveal something about the soul. It reaches into dimensions of depth the consciousness cannot get to. If the breath itself is used in a psychotherapeutic way, regulated by the laws of speech, it may uncover and dissolve even traumas that have already become fixed in the body.

Observe the breathing of a person who has just had a shock. The air is drawn in convulsively with a forced inhalation and is held. Never again may the person reach the same point of psychosomatic damming with his breath. He will do his best to avoid it by breathing in a more shallow or disfluent way. One may then observe how the person concerned will physically let out air when exhaling but withdraw emotionally at the same time.

There is a connection between free breathing and flowing body movement. As already mentioned, thought is immediately translated into activity through the speech organism during speaking. This ability to change from the pole of consciousness to the pole of life, which happens unconsciously

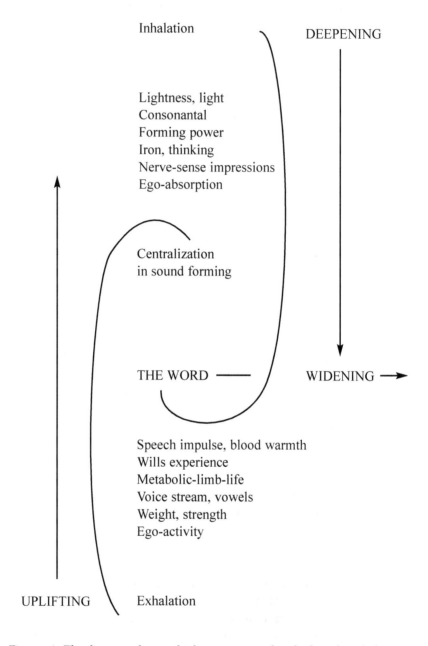

Figure. 4: The diagram shows which powers are absorbed on the inhalation and experience a deepening, and how with the exhalation the lower pole rises and experiences an uplifting. The inhalation adds something to people, the exhalation releases something. Both centralize themselves in the forming of the body.

Rateless ration
Roosted roomily
Reason wretched
Ruined Roland
Royalty roster

The **breath exercises** follow the articulation exercises and are designed to deepen the breath (first example) or to widen it (second example). In order to deepen the breath one needs to let go of the voice during the exhalation. In order to achieve a widening of the breath the inhalation needs to open up:

Deepening the breath: *Fulfilling goes*
Through hoping
Goes through longing
Through willing
Willing flows
In wavering
Wails in quavering
Waves veiling
Waving breathing
In freedom
Freedom winning
Kindling

Widening the breath: *In the vast unmeasured world-wide spaces,*
In the endless stream of time,
In the depths of human soul-life,
In the world's great revelations:
Seek the unfolding of life's great mystery.

The third group of exercises are for **agility of the speech**, resembling the so-called tongue twisters. Difficult sound combinations require the tongue to do gymnastics. This is also used in specific exercises for **sentence formation**. Fast and skilful consonant formation warms and enlivens the blood organism:

> *March smarten ten clap rigging rockets*
> *Crackling plopping lynxes*
> *Fling from forward forth*
> *Fling from forward forth*
> *Crackling plopping lynxes*
> *March smarten ten clap rigging rackets*

Only when voice and breath are proper in the consonants and can be supported by them, is it possible to work purposefully on the placement of the voice with **vowel exercises** and exercises for a correct placement of the voice. As soon as one learns to speak the vowels in accordance with its sound and not hastily, the breath will calm down. Part of this group of exercises are the dialogues between blood vowels (a, o, u) and nerve vowels (i, e), which are of particular importance for the therapy:

1. The quiet person:	*Marked you the pallor of that countenance?*
2. The nervous person:	*I didn't see anything strange in his face.*
1.	*You must look rather at what is crass.*
2.	*Take not my feelings of self from me.*
1.	*Hardly enough on guard are you.*
2.	*I will not take it that you say this!*

The remaining exercises are full of possibilities to train the speech qualities and grasp them in a differentiated way. The point always is to take hold of one's body in a new way with the help of the formation of the sounds, by casting off adopted, familiar and inherited speech habits. The differentiated sound forming capacity transforms the breath, and supported also through the articulation, frees the voice. Finding their own voice, the person has discovered something of their deeper self, in a comprehensive and wholesome way.

8.3 The Specific Therapeutic Approach

All the exercises given here have a regulating, hygienic effect. The numerous indications given by Rudolf Steiner, in the contexts of medicine and education, have been developed for use in therapeutic speech.

Through the breath the artistic means of speech becomes effective in the patient's body. He is consciously taught to contain himself in the articulation, to let go in his breath and to direct his voice.

Thus, the twelve syllable steps of the first articulation exercise *'Dart may these boats, through dark and leaves blowing'* (the two inbreaths each count as one step) can teach the heart patient to direct and regulate his heart beat better. The stepping of the syllables would then gradually be transformed into a rising rhythm, an iambic rhythm appropriate for the heart, alternating between short and long, contraction and expansion (systole and diastole), for example Wordsworth: 'I wandered lonely as a cloud...' Likewise the tongue can learn 'to step' with the help of the sounds D and T which have a consolidating effect on the restless heart:

Trip dauntless the door of doom.

Each exercise used therapeutically requires a particular construction, consisting of certain sound groups, rhythms, breath directions, gestures accompanying the breath, and poetic images. In this way it is possible to exert a very specific influence on the organism, provided the therapist has the appropriate knowledge and experience.

The aim is always to balance a particular one-sidedness that was diagnosed as related to the disease. Where there are tendencies of dissolution, a series of exercises may be used leading from blown sounds to impact sounds, via wave or vibrating sound, thus effecting consolidation.[59] Working in the opposite direction it is possible to loosen a certain hardening.

Depending on the area of the organism where a disorder is manifesting itself, appropriate sound groups are chosen according to the different placements. The lip sounds, for instance, have a particular effect on the front part of the human being to the upper abdomen. The tongue/teeth sounds, with their clear structure and radiating force, effect the back of the head and the spinal column. The palate sounds, on the other hand, have a warming (blown sounds) and moulding (impact sounds) effect on the metabolic-limb system.[60]

It is not always true that one heals a disease with the element opposite to it. Sometimes the similar element is required. Thus, for instance the blown or warmth sounds may be used successfully with inflammatory diseases, or the impact sounds with sclerotic illnesses, again, differentiated according to the three placements.[61] However, this requires that the patient practises in such a way that the blown sound is met with an inner strength and held back, while the impact sound is felt in its formative process. The decisive factor always is to research the different aspects of the speech remedies, using them in accordance with the needs of the person concerned.

In the therapy, it is not only the placement areas that matter but also the quality of the individual sound. While the voiced impact sounds (B, D, G) have a consolidating effect on the soul (astral body), the unvoiced impact sounds (P, T, K), the forming of which requires a lot of strength, mould deep

Anapaest:

The Assyrian came down like the wolf on the fold,
And his cohorts were gleaming with purple and gold;
And the sheen of their spears was like stars on the sea,
When the blue wave rolls nightly on deep Galilee.

                                          (From: The Destruction of Sennacherib, *by Byron)*

Dynamic speaking also has a therapeutic effect. An exercise as well as a sentence or a poem may be spoken with a faster or a slower dynamic. Working with longer or shorter pauses, questions and answers or throwing and catching a ball in different ways while speaking the soul experiences joyful mobility and liberation. In this way speaking is reinforced into the muscle organism and integrated into the person's feeling for movement.

Water poems starting at the lively source with the big stream finally flowing into the ocean are often good examples of a dynamic that is slowing down. The increasing dynamic always stimulates the will and thus the metabolism; conversely, in slowing down, a distance is achieved facilitating perception. The former has a more fuelling influence, the latter a more formative one on the breath and thereby on the organism.

The more differentiated one is able to experience the ways the different *styles* and placements are spoken, the more awakening they are. The person will be able in their speaking to take hold of their whole being more fully in thinking, feeling and willing. In the powerful *declamatory* poetry, for instance, such as alliteration, the breath penetrates deeply into the blood and will organism. Strong formative power and presence of mind are needed here.

In a rhythmical, *recitative* way of speaking, as for instance in the hexameter, the breath-blood-process calms down and a certain timelessness, a universality appears in the speech. A more detailed example of how to use these two styles in therapy is given in the chapter on neurasthenia and hysteria.

Directing exercises, as they are called, as well as some poetic verses awaken a feeling for the different soul qualities in thinking, feeling and willing.

Upward (feeling)	*Send thou upwards/yearning desire*
Forward (thinking)	*Send thou forwards/conscious striving*
Downward, backward (willing)	*Send thou backwards/conscientious reflection*

Mention must be made of the Adonis rhythm (– vv – v) which, due to its special combination of longs and short, brings about a strong harmonization of thinking, feeling and willing, or nerve-sense organization, rhythmic system and metabolic-limb system, respectively.

The gesture is a comprehensive revelation both of the speaker and the word spoken. In the beginning the gestures accompanying the speech follow the direction of speech and voice: by inhaling the patient learns to open up to the speech impulse coming from above, with the hands then following the speech downward. This movement may also be differentiated in a rhythmic way. The more the content is taken into consideration, the clearer the thought becomes — the gesture feels, points, describes, dissociates itself, etc. The following scheme shows the soul gestures revealed in speech, as given by Rudolf Steiner in *Speech and Drama.*[66] This basic description has since been further developed as a diagnostic and therapeutic tool.

Expression	Gesture	Quality of voice
1. Effective	pointing	incisive
2. Thoughtful	holding on to oneself	full-toned
3. Questioning	hands/arms rolling forward	trembling
4. Antipathy	flinging away of limbs	hard
5. Sympathy	reaching out to touch	gentle
6. Drawing back onto one's own ground	slanting limbs away from body	staccato, abrupt

The gesture is the most elementary way of learning how to incorporate and become the word, as it were, even into the body. Mime is a good example of this. In therapeutic speech the gesture is integrated into the speech process in such a way as to become audible in the voice.

Studying the gestures enables the human being to disregard himself, to lay aside his present 'role' freely slipping into another one. With this he can become more flexible in life situations, and strengthen his trust in the indestructible nature of the individuality.

Further examples of how to use the different therapeutic tools of artistic speech may be found in the case studies. For anybody wanting to follow the process of a therapy in detail it is necessary to thoroughly study the specialist literature given in the appendix.

Summary of therapeutic speech elements in exercises and poetry:

— Consonants — *according to their quality of solid, fluid, airy and warm; according to the three placements in the velar, dental and labial regions which correspond to the soul qualities of willing, thinking and feeling as well as the members of etheric body, astral body and ego.*
— Vowels — *according to their soul moods between widening and contracting, and their division into light vowels with a connection to the nerve-sense system and dark vowels with a connection to the blood.*
— Rhythm — *falling or rising, experienced in stepping and accompanying movements of the hand.*
— Dynamic speaking — *slowing down or increasing the speed.*
— Styles of speech — *epic, lyric, dramatic or recitation and declamation.*
— Gestures, role-playing — *based on the six archetypal dramatic gestures.*

CHAPTER 9

Neurasthenia and Hysteria
A Medical-Artistic Comparison

One of the most fruitful research activities in anthroposophical therapeutic speech is to compare artistic and medical descriptions given by Rudolf Steiner of the same basic phenomenon. One example is the polarity between the metabolic-limb organization and the nerve-sense organization (also called lower pole and upper pole of the human being, respectively).

9.1 The Medical Perspective

In March 1920 Rudolf Steiner spoke to doctors about neurasthenia and hysteria. This was at the beginning of his lectures to the doctors but comes up again and again throughout the lecture course entitled *Spiritual Science and Medicine.*[67]

The basis of a proper understanding of the polar functions taking place in the upper and lower pole of the human being gives insight into the true activity of the heart, which, according to Rudolf Steiner, is not the cause but the effect of the blood circulation. In this sense, the lower pole of the human being consists of any activity connected with taking in and processing food. Towards the upper pole these processes become more refined, as the blood approaches the activities of the nerve-sense system. This is where they encounter the breath, which may be understood as the lowest or least refined part of the activity of the upper pole of the human being. Here the exchange takes place between the food substances, which have been liquidized and transformed in the blood, and the air of the breath. This interaction is actually the essence of the middle part of the human being, or the rhythmic system.

'The polarity in the human being can only be understood correctly when one knows that man, as a dual-built being, perceives from the upper pole his lower pole.'

The organ of this perception is the heart.

too strong or the body is already weak. When the body is weak and there is prolonged imbalance, the ego-organization is no longer able at night to recreated the healthy balance in cooperation with the etheric body, and the result is severe somatic diseases.

9.2 The Artistic Perspective

Thoughts such as these which follow from the above-mentioned lecture course may lead to a description of the polarity of upper and lower pole of the human being, as given in the lecture course entitled *Poetry and the Art of Speech.*[69] These lectures were given six months after the medical lectures mentioned above. They are based on certain physiological principles of inhalation and exhalation.

When inhaling the diaphragm compresses the organs and vessels in the abdomen. These vessels in turn are connected to other finer vessels surrounding the spinal canal. This means that the pressure exerted on the blood vessels in the belly may easily make itself felt as a slightly higher pressure of the vessels in the spinal canal. This pressure is then passed on to the liquid which surrounds the brain. Thus, a pressure is created by the inhalation, the last waves of which reach the brain. To use a picture one might speak of a gentle touch.

The soul equivalent to this physiological process is the 'inhalation' of perceptions transformed into ideas with the help of the brain. Here, too, one may speak of a 'wave' which 'freezes' into idea. By joining the idea with a specific content of perception, the creative, living concept becomes fixed on the latter. This can be compared with the salt process — the crystallization of the concept. Thus, the inhalation movement can be characterized from two sides.

In contrast to inhalation, the exhalation is connected to the will. From a physiological point of view we can see the pressure wave described above flow back into the metabolic system after having reached the brain. In the healthy person it then carries insights from the upper pole of the human being into the realm of the metabolism and the will, where they are turned into action.

9.3 Recitation and Declamation

We have now reached the place of origin of two elemental polarities within the art of poetry: *recitation and declamation.*

To write recitative poetry means, in short: to take in an aspect of the world, 'digest' it inwardly and then bring it up again, re-cite it as poetry. To be more precise, what happens is that memory pictures rising up from the metabolic-limb system are held back in the middle sphere of the human being.[70] If they were not held back, the result of the process would be prose, which is closest to the quality of our ideas. In other words, recitative poetry is the result of a holding back in the middle sphere of memory pictures wanting to become ideas. Due to the quality of the middle sphere the pictures themselves are given rhythmical shape. This may result, for instance, in the hexameter as a living expression of the harmonic relationship of pulse and breath (4:1). But apart from the archetypal hexameter other rhythms may be the outcome; the whole gamut of metres is created, with either the element of pulse or breath prevailing. *'If we are dealing with the breath which is, as it were, counting out the beat within the blood circulation, we are looking at recitation. Recitation flows along in the harmony of the breathing process.'*

The following example of an hexameter is taken from *Andromeda* by Charles Kingsley.

Hour after hour in the darkness the wind rushed fierce to the landward,
Drenching the maiden with spray; she shivering, weary and drooping,
Stood with her heart full of thoughts, till the foam-crests gleamed in the
    twilight,
Leaping and laughing around, and the east grew red with the dawning.

Then on the ridge of the hills rose the broad bright sun in his glory,
Hurling his arrows abroad on the glittering crests of the surges,
Gilding the soft round bosoms of wood, and the downs of the coastland;
Gilding the weeds at her feet, and the foam-laced teeth of the ledges,
Showing the maiden her home through the veil of her locks, as they floated
Glistening, damp with the spray, in a long black cloud to the landward.

The Nordic people developed mainly the declamatory element of poetry. Here, it is the impulse to become active that is held back. Whenever the people of these regions were unable to make use of their strength in activities and fights, this strength was also held back in the middle sphere on its way into the will. This leads to a different kind of poetic element: alliteration. It is connected to the direction of the breath from the upper pole of the human being down to the lower.

'If it is the blood and what is blood-like by nature which sets the tone, if the blood imprints its strength, weakness, passion, emotion, tension and release onto the stream of the breath, then declamation results.'

The following example of alliteration is taken from *The Blacksmiths* (15th century English):

> *Swart smirched smiths smattered with smoke*
> *Drive me to death with din of their dents.*
> *Such noise on nights ne'er heard men never,*
> *Such clashing of cries and clattering of knocks.*
> *The craftsmen clamour for coal, coal, coal*
> *And blow their bellows their brains to burst.*
> *They jostle and jangle they jape and they jest,*
> *They groove and they grind and they grumble together,*
> *Hot with heaving of their heavy hammers.*

9.4 The Therapeutic Ideal

Let us combine the above elements to form an idea for the therapy. As mentioned above the neurasthenic person tends to produce too many ideas which may overstrain the head pole. At the same time there is a lack of *communication* with the lower pole: it is not perceived sufficiently. Here the speaking and experiencing of recitative poetry may be of therapeutic help. The content of what is perceived needs to be repeated and digested. Instead of turning it into prose it is recited.

At the same time the patient is taught to experience the metre, that is to say his breath connects with the rhythm of the pulse in a harmonious way. The heart is stimulated again to become the organ of perception for the lower pole of the human being.

In the hysteric person the relationship between will and outside world is subtly disturbed. Often he is stirred into activity by outside events or by unconscious emotions and drives. If this tendency prevails for too long, it leads to a state of hysteric exhaustion.

Here declamatory poetry may be helpful, for it holds the will back in the process of exhalation before it can become activity but forms that exhalation with ego-filled speech directed by the ego. It becomes immediately obvious if the intention in the upper pole is strong enough to really fire the processes of the lower pole. If it is not, there are ways of strengthening the declamatory forces with the help of certain exercises and texts. Damaging chaotic will force, easily affected by outer influence, is put step by step under the control of the ego.

In either case the therapist is thus working on the fundamental task of the rhythmic system, namely to bring about communication and balance between the upper and the lower pole.

9.5 Characteristics in Speech Diagnosis

Neurasthenic

General aspects
Enjoys working on a text for a longer period of time. Likes to speak after the therapist. Corrections may best be given by way of spoken examples and pictures. Therapy often goes on for many years, sometimes changing from pure therapeutic work into artistic work. Enjoys speaking in spite of difficulties. Slow to change. Sometimes stuck with word content.

Stance
Stiff, upright posture. In women there is a tendency to develop kyphosis in the upper thoracic spine. Stepping often stiff, but in general there is a better connection to stepping than to gesturing. Modified stepping difficult.

Often poor relationship to the directions of space: Hesitantly forward; fearfully backward; feeling between above and below limited; difficult to change between left and right. Narrowness.

Breath
The breathing as a whole seems to be narrow; there is no preferred type of breath. It is necessary to inhale slowly so as to make the breathing organism expand gradually. An important aim of therapy is to stretch the exhalation to the end of the phrase being spoken. Increasing the length by way of practising is very successful. Breathing exercises while sitting down are also helpful. Gently speaking on the lips and experiencing the sounds while accompanying the line with a gesture from above down helps to reconnect breath and pulse.

Voice
Tone usually normal to low. Voice seldom pleasant-sounding; little modulation. On demand, in repeating after the therapist, it can be loud but monotonous, undramatic. Very difficult to get a 'normal' emotional tinge into the voice. When trying it tends to become loud, unpleasant, even dragging. The voice easily reflects the person's state.

CHAPTER 10

Observations of Some Illnesses
with Case Studies

With the illnesses described below we will try to develop the diagnosis and therapy from speech and breathing phenomena, relating the former to Rudolf Steiner's 'knowledge of the human being.' In order to describe the approach taken in anthroposophic therapeutic speech, we have consciously decided not to include the explanations given by orthodox medicine.

The way people breathe clearly shows how closely interrelated the breath and the soul are, and that a merely physical, unensouled breathing activity is not sufficient to provide the human being with the feeling of buoyancy, the light radiance and the warming-through necessary for their health.

While the inhalation reaches into the space above and behind, the exhalation should be released into the space in front and below. Knowing this, it becomes possible to diagnose one-sided rhythmic processes as a disturbance of the relationship between body and soul, and treat them correspondingly.

The two different directions that the speech takes in declamation (breathe and speak from above down) and in recitation (from behind forward), are taught as basic elements of anthroposophic therapeutic speech (deepening and widening the breath). They may be used in a modified way, for instance in vocalic or consonantal speaking or in picture and rhythm. A further explanation of the significance of these styles is given in the chapter on neurasthenia and hysteria.

In the following, appropriate case examples are given to exemplify the concrete course of therapies.

10.1 Asthma and Depression: — A Comparative Breathing Study

The main difficulty of the asthmatic is his inability to exhale. This goes along with another inability, namely to let go of the consciousness pole (corresponding to inhalation) and give himself to the life pole (exhalation).[71] Therefore, the difficulty in breathing often increases when lying down since the horizontal position of the body places the human being in the more vegetative direction of space which threatens to deprive him of his waking consciousness. This often means that the asthmatic can only go to sleep while sitting up, since it is easier for him in the upright body position to cope with what oppresses him.

It is obvious that we are dealing here with fears rising up from metabolic processes that are neither formed nor worked through. The trigger may be an allergy. Often, however, the cause is undigested traumatic experiences.

In order to assert himself the asthmatic keeps himself awake artificially, evading the vegetative processes, as it were, letting the nerve-sense processes sink as far down as the exhalation.[72]

With regard to the breathing process this means that the asthmatic cannot find the etheric quality of the exhalation, that is to say the releasing quality. As a consequence the astral quality of the inhalation is transferred to the outbreath. The astral body then forms proper 'barbs' against the exhalation which may develop into the Charcot-Leyden crystals as far down as in the secretion of the mucous membrane of the lungs. This phenomenon is a clear manifestation of the formative force of the astral body. Due to the disturbed exhalation process it is not possible to breathe in a sufficient amount of air. The asthmatic person is in danger of suffocating since he is unable to rid himself of the used air.

Rudolf Steiner speaks of an insufficient 'switching point' between inhalation and exhalation, which prevents a change-over from the upper to the lower members.[73] The asthmatic is unable to exhale because he transfers the activity of the astral body and its alertness to the unconscious life processes of the etheric body. It is as if he was living with his consciousness shifted one floor downwards, but with no ground floor. This is confirmed by the phenomenon that in many asthmatics an attack may be triggered by merely thinking about certain things.

The very opposite is true for the breathing of the depressive who dwells in the basement, as it were, given over to heaviness, locked up in the physical body like in a dungeon, unable to find the way upstairs where he might find relief and a certain distance to his problems.

Here it becomes very obvious how a merely physical inhalation, which does not widen the soul while at the same time filling it with light and lightness, pushes the human being into heaviness. The inhalation is without inspiration and lacks an awakening, arterially stimulating character. Here it is the etheric, dull quality of the exhalation that is transferred to the inhalation leading to the corresponding soul mood of despondency and lack of drive.

When the depressive person inhales his astral body stays pressed together and therefore void.[74] Try to blow up a balloon compressed between your hands — that is the soul mood of the depressive when inhaling, unable thus to balance out the heaviness. He breathes himself 'downward' instead of 'upward,' so that the nerve-sense organism is also burdened and darkened, which consequently leads to negative compulsive thoughts. The lower pole prevails.

Both in the asthmatic and the depressive the rhythmic system is not in a position to fulfil its mediating function: the asthmatic cannot get down, the depressive cannot connect with the forces of the upper pole. In the former it is the nerve-sense process, in the latter the metabolic process which becomes the barrier blocking the rhythmic process and damming up the breath.

The task of therapeutic speech is to free the breath from these shackles and reintegrate it into the whole organism as a mediating link. With asthma the barrier may be overcome by means of strong declamatory exercises speaking from above downward, so that the over-alert consciousness may let go and transform into warming impulses of the will. This would, to a certain extent, correspond to an adrenaline therapy pulling the astral body down into the kidney system, thereby freeing the lungs. In a subsequent step the patient may be guided to a musically-released quality of exhalation by means of a type of inhalation adapted from the rising spinal fluid (as is the case in recitative speaking). In medical terms, this would correspond more to a copper therapy.

In the case of depression the opposite applies. In order to trust and open up to a new way of speaking and breathing, the patient first needs to break down his narrowness, his heaviness and rigidity, step by step widening himself by way of rhythmic recitation. Only then can he learn through a stretched inhalation how to widen upward — by seizing the speech very quickly as is typical for a declamatory way of speaking.

help to her was the beautifully balanced amphibrachys in the verse by Rudolf Steiner: '*Das Schöne bewundern ...*' Five-word /**e**/-exercises connected with stepping the pentagram to strengthen the ego in the etheric, in the solar plexus in particular: (*Lebendige Wesen treten wesendes Leben./ Lay bending various trays*).

Harmonization through the sounds by working on the transitions from H to M and from S to M, that is to say finding a way from the extremes (H = dissolution and S = sharpness) to the mediating M. After that many M exercises in order to give a smooth, loosening quality to the exhalation. Just as in the beginning with the sound B, the lip region was worked on once again: this time, however, not creating a boundary but giving oneself to the air.

Speaking dynamic sound sequences forward and backward in order to rearrange the connection between ego and world.

Poetry: Tree poems to imitate the bronchial 'tree' in the breath. Swinging poems (bell), alliteration to connect breathing and blood. Alternation of contracting and expanding texts and rhythms. Finally return to hexameter which the patient was then able to speak with a released and relaxed breathing rhythm.

4.1 Findings at the End of the Therapy
At the end of the therapy the patient had developed a new kind of stability. While during the first weeks she kept saying that she would not be able to cope with another crisis, she was now ready and willing to face possible new challenges and inner transformations. She had a positive attitude towards life and was largely free of fears. Her asthma was almost forgotten, she was less prone to infections, her organism was warmed through and taken hold of. She had developed a new attitude towards spiritual questions, which did lead to conflicts with her colleagues and a certain loneliness but the patient felt up to coping with them.

5.1 Comments and Therapeutic Suggestions
Suggestions for the future: Work consistently towards a living and spiritual thinking and let the results enter into your life and profession.

If the asthma should return, speaking and breathing habits need to be readjusted.

Case Study 2: Agitated depression. Male patient, aged 40, teacher

1.1 Period of Treatment
Forty-six therapy sessions of forty-five minutes each for eighteen months; in emergency periods daily practising together for about a week, twenty minutes per day.

2.1 First Impression
Patient looks dejected and given over to heaviness, movement and speech much slowed down. Due to the psychiatric drugs he gives the impression of being overconformist and 'soul-less,' but very willing.

2.2 Biographical and Medical Aspects
From the age of 21 severe agitated depression with manic phases. Congestion in the liver area, tension in the shoulders, flabby tissue. Disturbed sleep, constipation. Unfit to work due to diminished drive. After three suicide attempts admitted to a psychiatric clinic. Grandmother, mother and brother suffering from severe depression. His strong will to master his own fate is noteworthy.

2.3 Speech Diagnosis
Stance: Heavy body with sloping shoulders constricting the chest. Steps giving way as if the ground was not carrying him. Trying in vain to find a support.

Breathing: His inhalation was cramped having no enlivening, stimulating effect at all, since his soul remained compressed, unable to open up to the air. His exhalation was calm but without energy. Between exhalation and inhalation there was an empty moment, as if the patient needed to force himself to take another breath. No connection between breathing, sound formation and voice.

Voice: His voice was dark, slightly hoarse with the blood vowels /a/ /o/ /u/ prevailing.

Articulation: All consonants had the quality of impact sounds; they were formed rigidly and mechanically. Due to the psychotropic drugs his tongue (the soul's organ of touch) was sluggish and his mouth was dry. His lips became taut when forming the lip sounds M and B. M — the sound of the middle and of harmony — was the weakest sound.

Thinking: His thought processes had become independent, were going around in circles. There was either self-reproach or illusion. At the same time skilful use of language, great persuasiveness, but stereotype.

3.1 Therapeutic Aims

Make lighter what is heavy, move what has become rigid, bring light into the darkness. Incarnate the patient into lightness. Depression draws down, but speech gives uprightness from childhood onwards.

3.2 Course of Therapy

In little steps the attempt was made to get hands and feet out of the heaviness leading them into rhythmical movement. For this purpose impact sounds were used, which were in accordance with the way the patient was basically feeling. For the feet: *'Drück die Dinge die beiden Narrenkappen Tag um Tag'* (*Tricked deep dingle deep biting narrow copper dark too dark*). One step for each syllable. After that different rhythms (trochee, hexameter, choriambus). For the hands: *Bei biedern Bauern bleib brav'* (*By beaten bowers bide brave*) holding a copper ball in both hands. Then from feeling the rhythms with the hands gradually going into basic ensouled gestures.

Experiencing his own warmth by exhaling on H, then gradually leading the exhalation into a silent, streaming M. After that M-exercises, followed by increasing mobility with the help of the wave sound L and the vibrating sound R. R-exercises — also stepping backwards — were later used purposefully with the first signs of constipation which always preceded the depression.

Speech agility exercises were used to reenliven the tongue in order to make the soul active despite the psychiatric drugs. A new relationship was established between the vowels /i/ and /e/, between light and earth. Gradually the voice was enabled to stream on the exhalation by way of exercises involving rhythm, melody and gesture. Letting the voice stream out on the breath was experienced by the patient as a liberation of the soul from its incarceration in the body. (In his biography the Dutch psychiatrist Dr C. Kuiper says: 'What is the feeling of oppression — be it from fear, be it from depression — but the inability to breathe freely?') This means that the free breath is the healer of the depressed person, and the process of healing begins with an ensouled inhalation in which the person inwardly hears in advance the formative, ordering, liberating, awakening and purifying qualities the speech has to give. This filled the patient's inhalation with joy, also using gestures and the eyes to take hold of the upper space. The experience that the speech is streaming on the breath and is carried and supported by the air gave him courage and confidence.

As a constitutional exercise the patient was given an R-exercise:

Redlich ratsam	*Rateless ration*
Rüstet rühmlich	*Roosted roomily*
Riesig rächend	*Reason wretched*
Ruhig rollend	*Ruined Roland*
Reuige Rosse	*Royalty roster*

This exercise unites all the elements of his therapy.

4.1 Findings at the End of the Therapy

After a few months the psychiatric drugs could gradually be discontinued. Going through another phase of sleeplessness after nine months of therapeutic speech, the patient was able to cope without relapsing into depression. During this time he came for a daily practice period of twenty minutes.

He was then able to go back to work but returned regularly after the end of the therapy for a limited number of sessions. He experienced the speech work as an important help in his daily life, which he felt had reconnected him with his destiny.

5.1 Comments and Therapeutic Suggestions

After three years of inner and outer stability the patient gradually entered into a long manic phase, during which he broke off his contact with both his doctor and the therapist, since he experienced himself as well and healed. When he was hospitalized again during the following depression, he resumed the speech work.

10.2 Eating Disorders:The Soul's Refusal to Breathe its Way Down into the Body

Speaking and breathing relate to the process of eating. The organs that use the air are also involved in breaking up and tasting the food. Also the breath itself undergoes a metabolic process where it is taken in, transformed and excreted.

Thus, in all patients suffering from an eating disorder, a breathing problem may be diagnosed that has shifted to the metabolic system. Typical eating habits can be:

1) Too much or too little food is taken in (inhalation); **2**) Excretion of the food is induced artificially by vomiting or laxative (exhalation); **3**) The

2.3 Speech diagnosis

Stance: Careless, shuffling gait, ungrounded.

Breathing: Shallow breathing, filling only the upper part of the lungs, with shoulders pulled up and tense. Tense arms and legs. No connection to her own speech. Pushes it away, staying apart from it.

Voice: Dark and slightly tense.

Articulation: Weak blown sounds (F,W, S) showing a lack of warmth and direction as well as a lack of will for the lower part to treat the upper (hard front teeth on soft lower lip). Doesn't take on her own being (her speech). Articulation at first unclear; when corrected it is hard, disconnected. No sense of the sounds.

Thinking: Clear and rational.

3.1 Therapeutic aims

Build up uprightness from inside, take hold of the body with dignity. Stimulate the breathing metabolism, bring light into her inhalation, warmth into her exhalation, establish a connection between speech and speaker. Pay attention to the transformation processes taking place from in- to exhalation, and the other way round.

3.2 Course of therapy

Exercises were done to 'breathe' in and out heaviness and lightness through the knees, in order to stimulate her uprightness from below. Step the vowel sequence /a/ /e/ /i/ /o/ /u/, experiencing it from behind towards forward and feeling the curve of the foot in connection with the domed roof of the mouth. Experience the threshold of the lips by alternating between M (connecting with the air) and S (withdrawing from the air): *Mäuse messen mein Essen /Moisten mason mine essence.*

R-exercises to increase the breathing metabolism and reduce her fears. Directed gestures from far above going deep down. Exercises for the voice to fall into the breath step by step (*Erfüllung geht/Fulfilling goes*; Rudolf Steiner calls this 'finding yourself while letting yourself fall').[82]

The patient learns to orient her inhalation by what is to be breathed out, e.g. by long and short sentences, different rhythms and pictures. B-exercises to create support and a sheath in the belly region, which corresponds to the lip sounds, accompanied by round gestures.

The palate sounds G and K were practised to help the ego incarnate in the life processes (see Chapter 6 — 'Knowledge of the Human Being with regard to speech'). S-exercises, clearly formed at the dental placement, for newly grasped consciousness. Then on into the light nerve vowels /i/ and /e/, spoken in such a way that they may radiate light into the darkness. Forceful breathing out with the help of the blown sounds. Then on to the /u/. When the articulation was improved, the sounds were sensitively 'tasted' in different parts of the body, including the feet. After the word 'tasting' was mentioned the patient stayed away for a week — she had suddenly understood the connection between speech and nutritional processes. When she came back she made progress. Texts connected to the earth, first falling rhythms, then more and more rising ones. Stimulating the blood pole by means of fast sequences of consonants; later alliteration. Finally a dramatic scene from Goethe's *Iphigenie*.

4.1 Findings at the end of the therapy
When the therapy was finished the patient gave the impression that she was much more stable. Her eating behaviour was normal. In the meantime she has started a training course in speech formation.

10.3 Iron Deficiency Anaemia and Speech Processes[76]

All symptoms and troubles observed with iron deficiency suggest that the patients cannot seize their body sufficiently: conspicuous tiredness and a great need for sleep, poor efficiency, poor concentration, increased need for warmth, proneness to infections, and often a depressive mood combined with lethargy and weakness of will. The clinical symptoms include a pale skin and metabolic weakness. The speech is soft, weak, high or hoarse, often contrasting with the heaviness of the body. The inhalation is weak, with little impulse. The exhalation is stopped long before all the air is used up. On the whole the patient's speech and breathing lack in clearness and contour, their articulation tends to be slurred with minimal use of the speech muscles.

Rudolf Steiner's remark that by the strength of the voice one can tell whether a person has sufficient iron in the blood, obviously has a reference to these other symptoms as well. There seems to be a strong connection between iron and speech.[77]

Worth mentioning above all is the 'struggle of the iron' against the forces of the protein with its inherent tendency to cause illness and decay.[78] This is really a struggle of the forces of consciousness radiating into the human being from above and bringing formation, alertness and uprightness against the unformed forces of the body bearing down and bringing sleepiness.

This direction from above down, from thought to articulation, from inhalation to exhalation, is clearly the same as in the speech process.

A different connection exists between the kind of breathing deepened by 'inspired' speaking, which leads to a stronger intake of oxygen, and the role which the haemoglobin plays in taking in and distributing the oxygen. The iron gives the red blood corpuscles the necessary buoyancy, just as an organism well breathed through and formed by the power of speech lives in lightness. And both also affect the emotional well-being — depression often being related to iron deficiency.

With patients suffering from iron deficiency, the spirit-inspired inhalation, which is the basis of every true speech impulse, is of great importance in the therapy. In many cases it helped to improve the blood count immediately, particularly where medicinal treatment had been unsuccessful. Rudolf Steiner's observation may be helpful in this connection: '[the blood] is shot through, radiated through everywhere by what radiates into the blood as iron, not in as materialistic a way as today's science imagines but on the impulse of spirit and soul.'[79]

The patients' health will decisively be improved by stimulating their inner activity.

To get a deeper understanding of the true nature of the iron processes it is necessary to refer to the double sides of its nature. Iron makes up 4.7% of the earth's crust, or 47 kg per tonne of material. Less well known is that meteoric showers drop up to 10,000 tons per day into the Earth's atmosphere.[80] This fine meteoric dust is inhaled, and according to Rudolf Steiner provides the organism with its most important intake of iron.[81]

The decisive part of therapeutic speech is to increase the receptivity for this 'sun iron' by way of a deeper inhalation. If, with the help of the breath thus activated, the articulation is seized and the word moulded from above downward, the patient experiences the speech process as a recasting and transformation of his whole being.

Let it be pointed out that iron deficiency in particular appears in very different constitutions and will need differentiated treatment. In some cases the problem is not so much that not enough iron is taken in but rather that the iron is not transmitted to the metabolism. What is needed in this case is not just the impulse-giving speech forces but also thorough rhythmic work.

Case Study 4: Anaemia. Female patient, aged 33, mother of three

1.1 Period of Treatment
Nineteen months, with interruptions, on a weekly basis.

2.1 First Impression
Unformed, fairly coarse features. Round, heavy body (Gestalt), awkward, heavy gait, striking O-position of the feet. Although she had been living in the country for a long time, no relationship to the German language.

2.2 Biographical and Medical Aspects
From puberty iron deficiency, which had been treated in the US with massive doses of iron but without lasting success. Concentration problems, peripheral circulation problems. Started to study psychology when very young — during this time long depressive phase over several years.

2.3 Speech Diagnosis
Stance: Heavy movements, falling into heaviness.
Breathing: Shallow breathing rhythm with little impulse. Weak exhalation, shallow inhalation.
Voice: Muffled vowels. When speaking with more strength, her voice got stuck in her head.
Articulation: Unformed and slurred. Consonants pulled into one another, the foreign language not clearly understandable.

Processes of lightness/heaviness and light/dark disturbed.

3.1 Therapeutic Aims
Bring light into the darkness, make the heaviness lighter, give form to what is unformed, give warmth to the cold. Take hold of her body from above downward and shape it. Ensoul and stimulate her breathing.

3.2 Course of Therapy
In declamation, which is connected with the will, one can experience how the breath strikes the metabolism and works into the blood organism.[83] As a preparation for the declamatory style, the formative forces working in sound formation were practised, preferably with the well-suited five articulation exercises, moulding them in the breath-stream from above downward. In order to bring inner differentiation to the forces rising up and those working from above, questions and answers

Only slowly are thoughts put into words. There tend to be serious coordination problems when asked to accompany the speech with gestures or to step a rhythm. The hands are more likely to point back at the speaker than at the outside word. Soul qualities find no way to be expressed. The flow of speech may be halted, the voice monotonous, and although the articulation may be clear, it is awkward and rigid. The patient tends to take many new breaths (whenever a new element of speech is to be seized) and it appears that with every inhalation they withdraw into themselves.

It is difficult for the tinnitus patient to disregard or not to listen to himself, which means that he is condemned, also physically, to constantly experience himself. The ear, which normally devotes itself to the outer world, turns inside and transmits the sounds of the body which then drown out the sounds coming from the world and from other people.

The fact that he is thrown back on himself with the tendency to become a self-obsessed loner is what makes the Tinnitus patient a prisoner, trapped in the boundaries of his body and condemned to endure the sounds of his 'jail' like a torture, always listening inwardly, ever more compulsively. It was shown that temperament and character can have a positive or negative influence on the Tinnitus. To the extent that the patient succeeds in turning his attention toward the world, despite the harrowing ringing in his ears, he learns to control his illness.

For the therapeutic speech treatment the task is clear:

In speaking the patient is to be encouraged to listen more and more to how the sounds are shaped in the air (i.e. to listen to the outer world). The patient must refrain, even when articulating very actively, from taking a new breath before each word. Rather, the speech is to flow smoothly on the breath. The exhalation is to be prolonged and clearly directed outward.

The decisive healing factor, however, is to guide the voice to the different articulated placements, allowing the breath then to lift the sounds into space. From there it can be perceived. It can be heard by the ear of the speaker like a sound reaching the human being from outside.

Since one is used to hearing one's own voice transmitted mainly from inside through the eustachian tube, it takes great conscious effort to learn to listen to one's own voice from outside. One of the most intimate aspects of the human being, the voice, can become an experience of the outer world. The most outward aspect, the physical body, is heard by the tinnitus patient as noises from inside. This means that there is a complete reversal of conditions.

In order to make the patient develop this new hearing activity, it is helpful to have him play around with his voice, listen to it resounding in different spaces or vessels, as well as experiment with different directions, voice gestures and nuances. In the course of the treatment the voice itself will reveal when the patient has begun to hear into the space.

Interesting in this connection is the fact that the most successful cure of orthodox medicine so far is the Tinnitus-Maker, which creates broadband noise in the ear, drowning out and neutralizing the Tinnitus. While this is a technical means of helping the patient listen outwards, anthroposophic therapeutic speech tries to stimulate the patient's inner activity, thereby also addressing the underlying cause of the disease.

Case Study 5: Tinnitus. Male patient, aged 41, teacher

1.1 Period of Treatment
Thirty-two sessions of forty-five minutes each, once a week.

2.1 First Impression
The patient has very slow and sluggish movements; he has a certain air of darkness, heaviness, introversion. No clear eye contact. A brooder.

2.2 Biographical and Medical Aspects
For about a year the patient has suffered from increasing subjective noises in his ears, which he experiences as a kind of torture and extreme emotional distress. Suicidal thoughts. He tried in vain to get help from specialists, acupuncturists and psychological counseling. The medication given to improve his circulation has made the Tinnitus worse. He is desperately seeking insight into the disease since all of the examinations brought negative results. He suffers from flatulence and burping. His mouth is very dry. Moreover loneliness and emotional problems. Suffered a trauma when his youngest brother was killed in an accident at the age of twenty-eight.

2.3 Speech Diagnosis
Stance: Angular figure, stiff and slightly bent neck, heavy gait, slow movements. When using gestures his finger tips point towards his body. Very poor coordination of speech and movement. Clumsy when stepping rhythms.
Breathing: Although the patient cannot get rid of his breath when speaking, he takes a new breath after every few words.
Voice: His voice is deep but with little expression or melody.
Articulation: Very well formed but hard. Lip impact sounds are prevailing, forming a firm boundary to the outer world.

Thinking: He has problems to put his thoughts into words; his sentence structure is awkward. Many pauses, then slowly a new question rises up from below. Everything that should come out is held back.

3.1 Therapeutic Aims

The patient gives the impression of hiding in his body. The challenge is to help the body become an expression of the soul again.

In order to achieve this, the activity of the senses has to be directed outward. Express, address, breathe out and learn to listen to his own voice resounding in the room.

The misdirected air processes need to be regulated by the speech process. The body needs to be brought into movement through rhythm to become more permeable.

3.2 Course of therapy

The first step was to make the patient let go of his tensions. We started from certain movements accompanying the speech. Rhythmical swinging of the legs was accompanied by an up and down movement of the hands and heels:

Auf und ab	*Up and down*
auf und ab	*Up and down*
wallt die Welle	*Swells the wave*
schwipp und schwapp	*Splish and splash*
(Chr. Slezak)	*(English equivalent)*

This was followed by an exercise involving the back, alternating between bending and stretching with corresponding words. Moreover there was a gradual letting go with the help of a text aiming at turning his self-centred brooding into acceptance of his destiny:

Der dir	*The one who does*
Das tat	*This deed*
Will wohl dir tun.	*For you.*
Folg ihm	*Seek Him*
Er ist	*He is*
Der Christ.	*The Christ.*
(Anna-Iduna Zehnder)	*(English equivalent)*

On the first syllable arms and hands are coming down from above, on the second syllable a step is made, with the foot taking over the arm movement and letting go downwards.

Later dental sounds were practised in exercises, clearly directed outward:

> *Hist! Strategy stern ...*

and

> *Die silberne blitzende Spitze des Speers*
> *schiesst in die Erde (Chr. Slezak)*
>
> *(The silvery glistening tip of the spear*
> *streaks deep in the Earth)*

The breathing exercise *Fulfilling goes ...* shaking his hands out from above downward, as if to get rid of something. Certain exercises also with a ball in order to get eyes, hands, feet into movement.

The agility exercises were thoroughly worked with and in connection with them the text *Heinzelmännchen zu Köln* with their numerous different activities worked out.

For a long time the patient had a hard time expressing himself emotionally and imitating spontaneously. Although expression was what he was seeking, he failed repeatedly due to the forces dammed up inside him. Trying to speak and step a rhythm with increasing dynamic, his voice — otherwise strong — completely failed him for a few minutes. Again and again he would interrupt the outstreaming flow of words by too frequent quick inhalations, which meant that he was withdrawing into himself. Consequently we had to work slowly and carefully.

Only when the patient had developed more fluent and more directed movements of breath, voice and gesture did we start with more purpose to train his perception of his own voice, thus directing his hearing process outward which was focusing inward.

We worked with different vowel exercises in different sound spaces, for instance speaking into our hollow hands, a cupboard, a corner of the room, a receptacle, as well as at home in the different rooms. The following U/O-exercise, which sends the blood to the periphery, was particularly well suited:

> *Storm wolf roars forth through door and tomb*
> *Bold wolves bored through door and tomb*
> *Doom taught wolves bold through door and tomb*

This process was further supported by appropriate poetry which also focused on listening outwards, for instance *It is a beauteous evening, calm and free (Wordsworth)* or *Slowly, silently now the moon (de la Mare)*.

2.3 Speech diagnosis

Stance: Apart from the aspects mentioned under 2.1 the patient showed a certain stiffness in all her movements. She is very sporty and muscular, enjoys horse riding, skiing etc. While stepping she puts the heels down first, swinging her legs in a military fashion.

Breathing: Immediately conspicuous was her slightly increased shallow breathing which made me think at first of hyperventilation symptoms. In the beginning, when reciting, the patient tended to inhale hastily and dam up her flow of speech. She is familiar with breathing techniques from sports, but has no inner connection to the breathing process. She says she cannot understand her mother, who does yoga.

Voice: Her voice is firm with a slight nasality, normal register. When stepping the patient tends to overemphasize the vowels. Her voice is 'in harmony' with her overall appearance.

Articulation: Her spontaneous articulation is inconspicuous. After the holidays and similar phases of 'vegetative' emphasis, her articulation became noticeably slurred. In reciting she enjoyed strong consonants; she rolls the R beautifully.

Thinking: The patient expresses herself well but not in a very differentiated way. She speaks in very general terms about her condition.

The main symptom clearly is her shallow breathing, along with her tendency to dam up the flow of speaking in the vowel. On the whole she is talented and speaks nicely, with a somewhat singing intonation in her dialect.

3.1 Therapeutic Aims

Deepen her breathing, thereby hopefully decreasing the likelihood of epileptic fits by loosening the congested astral body downward and consciously directing the breath through speech.

3.2 Course of Therapy

a) *The Therapeutic Means*

The patient was given the following clear information. On the one hand we would work with the hexameter trying to influence her overall condition; on the other hand I would give her an exercise that was to be used purposefully in critical situations (trembling of hands). The hexameter chosen was *'Hoch zu Flammen entbrannte ...'* (English equivalent: *Over the mountains aloft...*) from Goethe's *Achilleis*, the exercise was the verse by Rudolf Steiner *'Ich trage Ruhe in mir ...'* (*'Quiet I bear within me ...'*). The hexameter was accompanied by quiet stepping, lifting the arms shoulder-high, then lowering them; the Steiner verse was spoken in three steps, internalizing the words more and more; the patient was sitting on a chair. This was later followed by the exercise '*In the vast unmeasured world-wide spaces* ...,' in a similar process, but in four steps.

A second sequence consisted of: *Name neat Norman; OM; Verse with many A and later O: After darkness mantles far/ Hark what asks the evening star/ Over ocean over all/ Open be to morning call; hexameter.*

A third sequence followed: *Hexameter; Nimm mir nimmer (Name me gnomes/ Vase soaked vestibule/ mitt tiling mittiles)/ Leicht lief letztlich (Light leaf let's leave/ Rush rolling radar glide/ mine moot much full)/ Fulfilling goes/AEU-KLSFM.*

After a break in the therapy one last sequence followed: *O dios hypsimelatron (Greek hexameter)/Abracadabra/Fulfilling goes/Hist! Strategy stern/Stormwolf.*

b) *The therapeutic process*:
The session always began with ten minutes of hexameter speaking. After the exercise '*Quiet I bear ...*' the patient from the beginning experienced a great heaviness of her limbs up to her eyelids, as well as an inner quiet that she would have thought impossible before. This exercise was meant for her to use whenever the inner trembling occurred. After the fourth lesson she told me that she had felt the trembling again when riding. She then spoke the first lines of the exercise, and the trembling disappeared. The same effect was achieved later with the other exercises *(OM, Fulfilling goes)*.

After one month of therapy the fact that this effect could be reproduced by the patient gave her new confidence, which made her enjoy the therapy very much. She learned ten minutes of hexameter by heart and practised regularly. In the second month she began to notice how shallow and high her breath was when she was working at the computer. She would then stand up, open the window and practise OM until her breathing was deep and calm again.

After five months of therapy she stopped taking medicine[84] when she was under stress, only practising her speech exercises to prevent the trembling. To begin with she had a lot of trouble with the exercise '*Fulfilling goes*' which was introduced around this time.

She began to take hasty inhalations again, damming the flow of speech in the vowels. Interestingly enough it became her favourite exercise after four further sessions.

Each time the effect was so strong that she felt like going to sleep. Around this time there was a motorbike accident outside her house one night, which upset her very much. She decided not to take any medicine but practise instead. She was pleased to find that she was able to calm herself down completely in this way. Shortly afterwards she decided to put the therapy to the test and stayed up until two a.m. The next day she felt a slight cramping, practised all her exercises, and had no problems all through the day, feeling normal tiredness in the evening. After eight months (twenty-eight sessions) we concluded the therapy for the time being, since the patient felt that the aim had been reached.

After another six months, during which no problems occurred and she practised whenever necessary, we added a series of ten refresher sessions at her request.

During this time she learned a Greek hexameter and worked intensively with the above-mentioned new exercises. After her skiing holidays she returned to her lessons sun-tanned and with a weaker articulation. What was conspicuous in the exercise *Abracadabra* was how difficult it was for her to speak the last line *Cadarabraba* with the necessary presence of mind and sharpness, to direct the force of the astral body outward. She compared it to trying to make a horse jump a fence, when you have to 'pull yourself together' in a similar way. As soon as she could muster the necessary presence of mind, there was 'Ego-presence' in her voice, too, while otherwise she would simply recite nicely out of her talent.

4.1 Findings at the End of the Therapy
Due to our work first in a pronounced recitative style and later with a more energetic exhalation the patient was able to experience her voice and breath consciously.

This was a completely new exercise for her. She learned to inhale without haste and direct her content-filled outbreath outward. This meant that the main symptom with regard to the diagnosis according to 2.3 had clearly improved. During the first period of observation of eighteen months she learned to prevent the fits in the initial stage by using an appropriate breathing technique. Later she did not practise any more and had three fits when returning from an exhausting holiday abroad.

She then came back into therapy, and had no more fits. A further control EEG at the University Hospital surprisingly showed no more epileptic activity. However, while the EEG was being taken, she had silently spoken one of the exercises regulating the breathing. When the neurologist compared the former EEG results with the new ones, the difference was confirmed. We believe that this is a clear proof mainly of the effect of the breathing exercise on her present condition.

With regard to the seven steps of the therapeutic speech process the patient on the whole reached levels four to five. At the end she mastered the exercises *Fulfilling goes, OM, AEU-KLSFM* with the confidence of level five, the hexameter of level four and the exercise *In the vast unmeasured* of level three.

5.1 Comments, Recommendations

Interesting in this case is the strong effect of the exercise *'Fulfilling goes ...'* after a few months' therapy, while in the beginning the recitative style of working was the right approach. This was logical from the speech point of view and dominated the whole therapy. The verification of the working hypothesis that the fits were due to congestion in the astral body, is also of interest. The latter came to expression in the fast and shallow, or high chest, breathing. The therapy had a very positive influence on the patient's breathing, and as a consequence the symptoms of trembling and fits disappeared. It was possible each time to establish that there was a direct causal connection between the disappearance of the trembling and the correction of her breathing.

The disposition of the patient suggests that it would be advisable for her regularly to polish up what she has learned in the therapeutic speech sessions.

Case Study 7: Tachyarrhythmia. Male patient, aged 56, sales representative

1.1 Period of treatment

Eighteen therapy sessions of forty-five minutes each, once a week.

2.1 First impression

The massive, heavy body gives the impression of a garment that is too big, unformed and which he has not really taken hold of. His force of articulation is extremely weak, his breathing strained, slowed down by the body, with side-noises such as wheezing and hissing. His deep voice does not sound very internalized: it is booming rather, resounding *around* the patient. There is no support whatsoever in neither sound formation or in his breathing, or in the way he uses his voice. Despite a certain heaviness the patient seems hectic and nervous.

2.2 Biographical and Medical Aspects

Seven years ago a complete collapse with exhaustion and paralyses on the left side. Since then tachyarrythmia, tachycardia with a falling pulse rate, along with panic attacks. Unable to breathe involuntarily, consequently respiratory distress and feeling of suffocation. Moreover: stomach cramps, weak kidneys, sciatica. Disposition for depression.

night, to relieve acute problems, such as arrhythmia or restlessness. Since the end of the therapy he has not had any symptoms. On the whole he gives the impression of having both his life and himself under control coping even with states of crisis.

5.1 Comments, Recommendations
As long as Mr A. is able to use the exercises successfully as a medicine whenever necessary, there is no need to continue the treatment.

Form drawing might be a good additional therapy for him.

Case Study 8: Angina Pectoris. Female patient, aged 80

1.1 Period of Treatment
Thirty-six sessions of thirty minutes each with a few breaks in between.

2.1 First Impression
Corpulent body, firm character, authoritarian manner. She talks too much and too fast.

2.2 Biographical and Medical Aspects
The patient repeatedly suffers from attacks of angina pectoris with breathing problems and chest pain which extends into her left arm. The resulting heart trouble was beginning to be very serious.

The medical diagnosis read as follows: heart failure (borderline compensated), diverticulitis, degenerative spine, as well as cataract.

2.3 Speech Diagnosis
Stance: Gestures as if beating time are interfering with the flow of speech.
Breathing: Her speech sounds hurried and breathless.
Voice: High-pitched.
Articulation: Although she speaks very fast, her articulation is clear.
Thinking: She has a tendency not to finish her sentences.

3.1 Therapeutic Aims
A calm but fluent way of speaking, interspersed with intervals, is to be encouraged, so that the strong and committed nature of the patient can follow and find expression for her rich world of ideas.

By acquiring a darker tone her voice should find more calmness; the flow of speech should not be interrupted by staccato gestures; keep up the flow of breath so as to relieve the heart.

3.2 Course of Therapy

Working with sentences consisting of monosyllabic words (*Dart may these boats...*) a certain regularity in speaking was achieved. The next aim was to harmonize the ratio of pulse and breath with the help of exercises spoken with four syllables on one breath:

> *Rateless ration*
> *Roosted roomily*
> *Reason wrechted*
> *Ruined Roland*
> *Royalty roster*

Followed by two hexameters:

> *(— Mile after mile through the meadows.....*
> *— Warm are the winds in the woodlands....)*

In order to strengthen the heart the sound /**a**/ was practised, both individually and in exercises and poems. The formative force of this sound can give structure to the whole human being. Later we worked with the iambic rhythm, which may be understood as a rhythm of the heart, e.g. in the fairy tale of the good and the bad by Rudolf Steiner.

To refine her breath we worked with the loosening sounds **M** and **L**, which have a positive effect on the cataract as well. This led us into the fluid element — falling in drops, rippling or flowing quietly — which the patient could experience in many different ways in exercises and corresponding examples in poetry.

To strengthen her uprightness we worked with speech exercises affecting the posture, such as bending and stretching with **R** and **K** (*'Mit dem Rücken kann ich mich bücken...'[With my back I can roll over]*). Secure and directed stepping was practised with the help of the following exercises: *'Genesen werden stets edle Seelenwesen'(The grey day breaks, breaks the grey day...)* and *'Wirre Würfe werfen wir würdig weg' (Virile viewer vividly vociferates vowels).* This had a positive effect also on the constitution of her back.

4.1 Findings at the End of the Therapy

A generally liberating and relieving effect had been achieved, also widening her chest. Whenever there was a sudden attack of angina pectoris the patient was now able to help herself with familiar exercises.

She has gained control over her voice, which is now pleasant to listen to and has a soothing effect.

She can continue to give courses in spiritual science, which is a considerable achievement at her age.

5.1 Recommendations
After an interval of six to twelve months if would be advisable for the patient to return and take a look at the way she practises on her own.

Case Study 9: Breast Cancer. Female patient, aged 62, retired teacher

1.1 Period of Treatment
October 1996 to October1998

2.1 First Impression
The patient is tall and slim, single, with grey hair and blue eyes, sixty-two years old. She seems reserved and polite. Immediately noticeable is her slightly broken, high voice with little modulation. Part of the time she is very short of breath and, in the first lesson, very nervous. She says she wants to 'try out' what speech formation is. On the whole, an inner impedance is prominent of everything fluid.

2.2 Biographical and Medical Aspects
The patient is a retired teacher. She used to be prone to depression; periodically she suffers from sleeping disturbances. It is difficult for her to let go. She tends to hold on to people and things, even when it is time for a new theme in life. She is sensitive to changes in the weather and is grumpy in the mornings. At the age of fifty-eight a lump was discovered in one of her breasts which was diagnosed as a breast cancer and operated on. There is a case of cancer in her immediate family. In her rhythmic system the astral body does not reach out sufficiently, consequently taking hold of the physical and etheric body in a way which causes disease. This region is not warmed through by the ego.

2.3 Speech Diagnosis
Stance: Tall and upright figure with a reluctant gait. What is conspicuous above all is how little connection she has to the directions in space. She seems to be withdrawn into herself. The backspace is as if cut-off; she has very little will-power to move forward. In the above-below, a forced uprightness is dominant, and the interplay between height and depth cannot unfold freely. With regard to right and left she limits herself to narrow

considerations; a broad-minded view, which she would be capable of assuming, is not fired with inner enthusiasm. The inability to reach out into the different directions of space with ensouled gestures, is typical of patients with breast cancer.

Breathing: At times there is shortness of breath, which has functional reasons, as well as shallow breathing. She has a long upper body and a good breathing volume. What she needs is to really widen her inhalation and gain strength from a deep exhalation.

Voice: Her voice is hoarse and held back with an unpleasant hardness to it whenever she speaks louder. However, the hoarse tone is due to constitutional reasons and often disappears with the correct breathing technique. Any ill-feelings immediately affect her voice.

Articulation: She has a tendency to over-articulate. Strong, hard impact sounds. Problems with voiced consonants and with the rolled R, although in her local dialect the R is usually rolled.

Thinking: She thinks about questions and problems for a long time before reluctantly expressing them.

3.1 Therapeutic Aims

Widen her in all directions of space with the help of speech which she should learn to take hold of in a feeling way. She needs to learn to experience herself as a rightful inhabitant of the space around her, radiating her desires and will impulses by means of gesture and speech. Free her voice from its constriction in the breast and larynx area by deepening her inhalation and strengthening her exhalation. Hearing her voice resound outside of herself could also be a means of experiencing herself from outside as an ego-endowed being.

3.2 Course of Therapy

a) *Therapeutic Means*

With the help of different sequences of exercises we tried to widen and deepen her inhalation backward and downward. To begin with, her exhalation was connected to the feet by stepping, trying to bring this connection into a flowing movement. This was followed by exercises to make her experience her voice resounding in space. (The text used was the first bible translation into medieval German, with alliteration: *Heliand*.) A very helpful exercise in the beginning was: *Sprache-sprechen-spritzen-sprossen-sprudeln (Sparkling-spraying-speaking-spoken-sprucing)*, the syllables of which, after a deep inhalation, were directed forward while stepping them, each time speaking one word more on the same breath. *Brause prächtig prunkend/ Durch das dortige*

2.2 Biographical and Medical Aspects

From birth the patient has suffered from kyphoscoliosis. When he was thirty-eight old his spine was straightened surgically, and he was in hospital for many months. Although there was a certain improvement, and despite the medical treatment, he still suffers from considerable shortness of breath with the slightest physical exercise. This means that for two years he has been dependent on oxygen treatment for about sixteen hours every day. The treatment helps to more or less compensate for the restrictive disorder of ventilation caused by the spine. Even during the day he suffered from a compulsory need to sleep. Consequently a sleep apnoea syndrome was diagnosed and he will have to wear an oxygen mask with light excess pressure at night, too.

He suffers from masked depression with a tendency to agitation and occasional anxiety. His vital capacity is 49% of the norm.

He had to give up several professions and has received an EU-pension for the past six years.

Although the patient lives a secluded life he is not lonely and does not complain of his fate. He travels all over Europe in his caravan (camper van), swims and plays skittles.

2:3 Speech Diagnosis

Stance: Round back, bent over. Stiff neck.
Breathing: His breathing was congested, held back. The patient constantly has the feeling not to get enough air which causes fear.
Voice: His voice sounded pressed, stuck in the throat.
Articulation: His sounds were slurred, individual syllables were being swallowed.

3.1 Therapeutic Aims

Strengthen his own breathing so that he is able to help himself in distressing situations, and that the oxygen treatment may be reduced or possibly even discontinued. The fears caused by the respiratory distress are to be overcome and his self-esteem is to be strengthened. The recurring stiffness of the neck is to be removed.

3.2 Course of Therapy

With the help of certain exercises it was possible to activate his breathing in such a way that the patient's will to live was strengthened and his respiratory distress was overcome. The exercises were chosen for the way in which the rhythm and the sounds, for instance Amphimacer (— ⏑ —), /**u**/, **V**, and **L**, are suitable to stimulate the exhalation, emptying the lungs as much as is needed for a new refreshing inhalation. These exercises were accompanied by suitable movements of the hands and arms, letting go of the lengths downward.

Practising the unvoiced blown sound **CH** (as in the Scottish **Loch**), which gives an experience of the movement and warmth of the breath in the mouth, helped the patient in situations that made him get out of breath (e.g. climbing stairs).

Schooling his voice with different vocalic exercises gave him new confidence in his own strength establishing a new self-esteem. We worked on the following vowel sequence in particular: **a, e, i, o, u**, accompanied by appropriate gestures, combining the vowels with different consonants (**Da De Di Do Du, Ta Te Ti To Tu** etc.) and letting them be released on the exhaled breath.

Towards the end of the therapy the velar sounds **G** and **K**, which challenge the breath and the will-force, as well as the sound **NG**, which can widen narrowness, were helpful to overcome his fears. **N** and **R** contributed to relaxing the cervical vertebrae in the shoulder area:

> *Narrow wren*
> *Mirror royal*
> *Gearing grizzled*
> *Noting nippers*
> *Fender coughing*

4.1 Findings at the end of the therapy

After two years of therapeutic speech his vital capacity had increased to 70% of the norm. During the day he does not need the oxygen treatment any more. Cortisone could be discontinued. His general condition had improved and he was able to experience himself in a new way. His spontaneous articulation also improved clearly. His breathing is no longer pressed or pushed, he no longer suffers from respiratory distress. Speech formation has become a much appreciated activity in the life of the patient.

5.1 Recommendations and Suggestions

The patient is able to help himself independently in situations of distress with certain exercises. He returns regularly for a period of weekly sessions in order to stabilize and/or improve his physical and emotional condition at the level he has reached.

Case Study 11: Colitis. Female patient, aged 43, housewife

1.1 Period of Treatment
Twenty-two sessions of thirty minutes per week. Later several refresher sessions of various length. Period of observation five years.

2.1 First Impression
Reluctant person with wooden movements. Her speech seems to cling to her, she opens her mouth only a very little. Says that she has come because the doctor has sent her. A very reserved person.

2.2 Biographical and Medical Aspects
The patient has great difficulties to set boundaries. Her husband always seems to complain that the household is a mess, although she is a very orderly person. She has severe problems in making decisions. In her first year at school she was hit on the knucklebones whenever her pronunciation was not correct. As a consequence her relationship to speech was disturbed to begin with. Hysteric constitution. From the age of thirty onwards, after her first child was born, the patient began to suffer from repeated diarrhoea. For a long time there were no pathological changes in the colon. At the age of forty a sub-acute ulcerative colitis was diagnosed. After another three years a severe-relapse with blood-stained diarrhoea and weight loss of eight kg. She was hospitalized in the Ita Wegman clinic. First contact with therapeutic speech. Medication: Salofalk and anthroposophical preparations. She also developed anaemia which was a further indication for the doctor that she should do speech formation.

2.3 Speech Diagnosis
Stance: Stiff, upright, reluctant stepping. Careful observer, distrustful. Steps rhythms in a stiff, military way. Finds gesturing difficult. Her limbs are 'alien' to her.
Breathing: Disfluent, shallow breathing with little power. The breath is not able to take hold of her speech and take it along.
Voice: Unmodulated, monotonous. First breathy, later at therapist's request uniformly loud. She does not experience anything when reciting herself, only when listening to speech.
Articulation: To begin with all consonants were weak. Her poorly formed lip sounds were striking. For a long time she formed the V incorrectly, that is with both lips.

Thinking: Contrast between a very differentiated perception of speech (in Italy she intoned like an Italian, she said) and a very poor memory for speech. Her connection to the etheric body seemed to be disturbed. On the whole an intelligent, differentiated person.

3.1 Therapeutic Aims
Offer her a new possibility to connect her speech (and thus her soul) with her body. This is to help her learn to set boundaries to her husband. Strengthen the astral body so that it can regain its healthy polarity in the body, together with the ego organization, and put an end to the dissolving activity in the metabolism. In terms of speech this means to experience the voice as a means of expressing her self with the help of the consonants. Return width to her breath.

3.2 Course of Therapy
The therapy basically proceeded in two directions:

During the acute episode a formative, moulding way of working with the following exercises:

Dart may these boats through dark and leaves blowing.
Gaunt crooked crummy Christmas logs can men cover.
(Constitutional exercise)
Kurze knorrige (Curtsey ignoringly...)
Come crooked craftiest cur.

These exercises were accompanied by concentrated gestures done close to the body and corresponding steps. Putting the hands on the hips and feeling into the pressure while speaking 'Gaunt crooked...' proved to be particularly effective. With the help of this exercise the patient was able, after the first series of sessions, more and more quickly to get control over the acute episodes of colitis which used to occur at times of emotional stress. In the observation period of five years the acute episodes became less and less frequent. With the first signs of severe diarrhoea she would begin to practise the exercise and was able to slow down the dynamic of the episode increasingly faster. Since then she no longer needed to consult the doctor because of colitis.

The second way of working consisted of a strong and radiating type of exercises, designed to strengthen the patient's stamina and ability to set boundaries:

alcoholic. The new father used to beat up the whole family. Her mother later died of an atrophy process in the brain.

At the age of nineteen stomach ulcer, anxiety, fits of rage. At the age of twenty-two first hospitalization in a psychiatric clinic. Later frequently readmitted.

At present she is a single mother (unable to work), suffering from a chronic subjective state of exhaustion. She needs a lot of sleep. No organic results. Anorexic behaviour.

2.3 Speech Diagnosis

Stance: Leptosome build, weak posture.

Breathing: The breath finds support neither in the body nor in the articulation placements, and consequently does not go very deep.

Voice: Her voice sits far back, with a dark colouring and strength which is hardly audible in her everyday speech.

Articulation: Very weak consonants.

Thinking: Her attitude basically seems to be sceptical and reluctant.

3.1 Therapeutic Aims

Strengthen her personality and/or will in order to allow the strength she really has to become effective.

Work on supporting the sound with the help of the consonants. Bring about a feeling of security by clear articulation and by working with lip sounds strengthening the ego (see Chapter 6 on the four bodily members of the human being) and helping to set boundaries.

3.2 Course of Therapy

At the beginning exercises for a better orientation in space — above/below with the verses:

Auf und ab	*Up and down*
auf und ab	*Up and down*
wallt die Welle	*Swells the wave*
schwipp und schwapp.	*Splish and splash.*

For backwards and forwards:

Hin und her	*To and fro*
hin und her	*To and fro*
fährt das Schiff	*Goes the ship*
übers Meer.	*Over seas.*

This was followed by dynamic speaking to liberate her soul from the different anxieties (see Chapter 6.3, **The Five Effects of Speech Development**). Practising the palate blown sound **CH** (like in the Scottish 'loch') and experiencing her own strength of breath, the patient was able to identify more strongly with herself. The voiced consonant **V** stimulated her own inner strength (vibrating the lower lip), step by step leading it outside. This was followed by the vowel sequence: **a**ch, **e**ch, **i**ch, **o**ch, **u**ch. This gave support and order to her soul.

Her strong need to yawn when speaking (a sign of her hunger for air) could be checked with the help of the impact sounds **M**, **K** and **B** with corresponding exercises. Gestures or stepping supported the strength to make these sounds, which were then brought into movement with the flowing **L**.

The sound /**u**/, which is particularly good for stimulating the peripheral circulation and brings ego presence to the lips, gave the patient courage and grounding (accompanied by gestures and feeling with the feet). With the help of **u**-exercises she learned to give herself support and strength in particularly difficult situations (for instance after a long drive). Moreover, this sound helped to improve her sleeping problems.

A new quality of balance, which the patient would not want to miss any more, was created by working on the text 'In the beginning was the word...' which was spoken line by line forward and backwards, ultimately just thinking the lines silently.

A declamatory, alliterated text (**M** and **L** prevailing) gave the patient new confidence in the power of the speech to carry her.

Her anxiety was reduced working with the sound **NG** in words she chose herself.

4.1 Findings at the End of the Therapy
The patient has learned to help herself with certain sounds and exercises, which she uses intermittently during the day to keep the forces generated by speech alive. She also has become aware of the necessity to conserve these forces.

5.1 Recommendations and Comments
If the patient takes further lessons every now and again and practises consistently, she will be able to strengthen herself and gain new soul and life forces that will carry her and enable her to keep developing.

Case Study 13: Vocal Nodules. Male patient, aged 37, architect

1.1 Period of Treatment
January to October 1997, thirteen sessions of thirty minutes each.

2.1 First Impression
The patient is about two meters tall, slim, his haircut is in the 'Che Guevara' style, he is well-groomed. He says that he does not know anything about this kind of therapy, but since his doctor recommended it, he has decided to give it a try.

2.2 Biographical and Medical Aspects
The patient is thirty-seven, happily married, no children. He is an architect in a joint office with other architects. At present he is without commissions, which means that he is *de facto* out of work.

Medical diagnosis: Vocal nodules, that is to say a hardening on the vocal chords which bother him when speaking. Having been removed by surgery, they reappeared very quickly. Prognosis: Irreparable. Accompanying symptoms were hoarseness and a certain inhibition during conversations.

12.4 Speech Diagnosis
Stance: There seems to be a disfluency in the area of larynx and collarbone; his head is slightly bent back, as a consequence the chin is slightly protruding; his shoulders are slightly pulled forward. In contrast to this, his arms and legs appear to be loose and relaxed.
Breathing: When the patient speaks it sounds as if he is holding his breath.
Voice: Sonorous, 'stuck' way back in his throat.
Articulation: His articulation is not formed, not at any of the placements. This gives the impression of purely vocalic, sonorous sound.
Thinking: The patient expresses himself in a simple but clear way.

3.1 Therapeutic Aims
Short-term: Lure his voice forward. Activate his exhalation in speaking. Make him seize his limbs harmoniously. Find support in articulating.

Medium-term: Relieve the strain on the vocal chords by practising regularly.

Long-term: Stabilize this 'relieved' way of speaking and transfer it to his everyday language.

3.2 Course of Therapy

a) *The Means of Therapy*

The patient is willing to practise by himself, which is a necessary prerequisite since he can come once in a fortnight only, the journey taking him five hours altogether. Due to unexpected professional commitments there were often two to four weeks between individual sessions.

1. A basic constitutional exercise was stepping the hexameter with arms coming down while speaking (approach with neurasthenic patients). Taking hold of the limbs in speaking; activating the breathing.
2. *Pfiffig pfeifen ...(Piffling fifer)* a) with the tip of the toes on every **pf**; b) with an arm gesture. These two ways were to be practised which the patient did *very* intensively. To balance out he also practised the exercise gently from the eighth session. We started with the first stanza of the exercise, gradually including also the other two. Focusing on the **pf** also made it possible to activate the labial placement (lips).
3. *Wuchtig wogt Wirbelwind ...(Warning warblers wallow weightily)* B while bouncing a ball. To further support the labial placement and activate the exhalation.

Sequence from the 8th session:

1. Hexameter
2. Pfiffig pfeifen...*(Pifling fifer)*
3. Zuwider zwingen...*(Tu-whit twinkle 'twas)* (with arm movement)
4. Halt hebe hurtig...*(Halt! habit hoarding)* (stamping in a standing position)
5. Wuchtig wogt...*(Warning warblers)*/ Pfui, pfeife pfiffige...*(Fie, fifer fifing)* (bouncing a ball)

In the second part of the therapy session we would do various exercises to fully grasp the different placements: Protzig preist...*(Proxy prized)*; Tritt dort...*(Trip dauntless)*; Marsch schmachtender...*(March smarten ten)*.

b) *Therapeutic Process*

To begin with the lip placement was seized actively, followed by the tongue/tooth placement and then the palate placement. This went along with activating the exhalation in speaking and directed movements of the arms and legs.

The patient practised regularly, diligently and consistently. At a certain worked on, the patient said that this was opening up a whole new world to her. She developed a good sense of humour during the sessions, and was always looking forward to them. She herself started to roll up her long sleeves. The fixed gaze of her eyes had disappeared, and she was no longer holding the palms up. She started to copy texts into her own little book and freely recited a different verse every week.

4.1 Findings at the End of the Therapy
After two months of treatment with therapeutic speech her eye pressure was stabilized despite continuing emotional stress.

5.1 Recommendations
She might profit a lot from the task of closely observing the weather every evening. In addition it would be advisable for her to continue with the speech.

Case Study 15: Dry Maculopathy. Female patient, aged 62, secretary

1.1 Period of Treatment
Forty-four sessions of thirty minutes each, once a week.

2.1 First Impression
The patient is small and round, well-groomed. She says she does not have any idea in which way speech might help her, but she has decided to come anyway since the doctor will know. She is very polite, conformist, unable to set boundaries to her grown-up children. She is afraid that she might go blind.

2.2 Biographical and Medical Aspects
Referral note from her doctor:

Maculopathy is caused, in general, by a disturbance of the strict separation of blood and nerve in the eye. The Saturn process in the eye is out of order. Describing the Saturn process here with all its consequences would go beyond the scope of this exposition. Like no other therapy, therapeutic speech is able to improve the ego and astral organization's free use of this sense organ. With regard to the organs, this means that the organism is enabled to strengthen this separation again. As a consequence, the function of retina and kidneys are improved to the extent that the outer light can be met by a more powerful inner light. This particular patient, who has a hysteric constitution, was suffering from a dry maculopathy, the inability to set boundaries against the outer world, as well as diabetes mellitus.

2.3 Speech Diagnosis

Stance: Poor coordination of speech and movement. Her hands are bent inwards.

Breathing: Short breath.

Voice: Monotonous, low, hard, chopped.

Articulation: Often not conscious. All consonants have the quality of impact sounds. She is not able to form **R**, **L** and **M** well.

Thinking: The patient's concentration is very poor. She does not like learning things by heart. Often it is necessary to stop her flood of words.

3.1 Therapeutic Aims

Stop the progressing maculopathy. Help her to set boundaries and strengthen her ego.

3.2 Course of Therapy

We worked, above all, with the basic speech exercises (articulation, breathing and agility exercises) which helped her to gain better control over her speech instrument and bring form and order into her speech. We also worked on objective, lyrical poetry.

Later we did the following two exercises:

— *R*ichtig recht rechnen *(Richly rigged rigging...)*
— *Bei meiner Waffe (By miner wafer...)*

Soon she was able also to form the exercise *Hum Ham Hem Him* well on the breath. As with most macula patients, in her case, too, the ball went zigzagging through the air when she threw it. She very much enjoyed stepping forwards and backwards on speech exercises.

After a while she started to follow her own interests instead of always being there only for the family.

4.1 Findings at the End of the Therapy

At the beginning of the therapy there was a chronic macular oedema which dried up. Since then her sight has remained the same. The diabetes is well stabilized.

5.1 Recommendations

Continue with therapeutic speech and the medicinal treatment.

CHAPTER 12

Typical Speech Disorders, their Assignment to the Articulation Regions and Therapy

As already mentioned briefly,[85] *therapeutic speech formation divides the speech organs into three main areas: labial (lips), dental (teeth/tongue) and velar (palate). These three areas may be regarded from the point of view of physical body, soul and spirit. Based on the knowledge of the human being, speech disorders as well as certain diseases and problems of the speech organs are to be related to these three main areas in the following chapter.*

To begin with let us compare the division of the consonants, as used in speech formation, according to the quality and way of formation and place of formation with the division used in general. Speech formation also distinguishes five **articulation regions** *which, however, are not fully identical with the customary ones, since the division of the speech organs is regarded as a reflection of the human being as a whole.*

In speech formation a qualitative assignment of the consonants to the elements (earth — impact sounds, water — wave sound, air — vibrating sound, fire — blown sound) is added to the usual division, according to the type of formation.

12.1 Labial (Lip) Region

The lips are a unique entrance and exit to the interior of the body. Formed by an orbicular muscle (Orbicularis oris) and embedded into the orofacial muscular system, which is innervated by the lower branch of the facial nerve, they are very sensitive to temperature differences. This means that they act as first guardians rejecting food or drinks which are too hot or too cold. They let in only what has been thus tested. They also open to let out the breath and the formed breath (speech), respectively. In doing so, they share in forming the lip sounds.

In the course of life the form of the lips changes in a very particular and characteristic way. While in babies and toddlers the upper lip still has the characteristic M-shape, showing like an open curtain their wonder of the world but also their total defencelessness, after the age of three something like an expression of the personality of the child begins to develop which ideally will culminate in a well-balanced upper and lower lip around the middle years.

In old age one-sidedness of the soul often comes to expression in the shape of the lips. As a rule, for instance, the lower lip is sticking out while the upper lip recedes. According to Rudolf Steiner, an expression of one's personal destiny is concentrated in the lower lip. Looking at different portraits (e.g. Goethe, Beethoven etc.) is very telling in this context.

This will show what it is, above all, that forms the shape of the lips in the course of life: our feelings. This is most obvious in babies. Sucking at his mother's breast he 'loves himself into the world.' At this stage the baby's love is nothing but need for food. The sucking movements lay the basis for his own self-perception, which will come to expression in the correct closure of the lips at the end of the first year.

The therapy of orofacial dysfunctions, which recently has been the recipient of increasing attention, therefore speaks of 'incompetent lips' when the mouth is always open. This attitude has often been observed in bottle-fed babies.

When the sucking movements have led to a sufficient maturation of the brain and, from an emotional point of view, the first physiological desire has been satisfied, there comes a time when the lips are steadily shaped, which climaxes around the age of twelve. Then the new desires that spring up, and the need to seize and shape these forces, again come to expression in the lips. The often distinct bulging of the lips during puberty reflects emotions such as defiance, rejection, or a great longing. At this time the basic shape is still very much determined by heredity. Entering into maturity is again characterized by a stronger balance of the lips with the whole shape of the face. Thus, it is possible in a beautiful way to follow how the personality incarnates into their body through different levels of intensity of love by observing the lips. In the second half of life, the lips become an expression of how the personality deals with their inner life and confronts themselves with the outer world.

In the red lips the colour of the blood comes close to the periphery. The colour of the lips gives clear information about the peripheral blood circulation. Pale or bluish lips show that the periphery is not sufficiently supplied with blood, as in shock, faint, coldness, etc. In all of these instances the ego does not feel at home in the world any more, and therefore pulls the blood back into the centre. An ideal of beauty in the fairy tale is: 'as white as snow, as red as blood and as black as ebony.' Red is the colour of the lips when the person is fully present in their body and thus attractive. With a kiss it is possible to meet ego to ego in the lips.

What was mentioned previously regarding the function of the lips as a guardian between inside and outside, also in a physical sense, applies likewise in a subtle way to speech. Two important emotional qualities — sympathy and withdrawing on one's own ground/setting boundaries — is expressed in the function of the lips. Everybody is familiar with the way the emotions play on the lips, within the whole range of facial expressions. Moreover, the lips are both a boundary and a connection between above and below. The lower lip is more significant in terms of the personality. 'In the muscles of the lower lip we have an intense concentration of our karma, of that karma that is so mysteriously present within us all the time.'[86]

Looking at the speech organs according to their assignment to metabolism, rhythmic system and nervous system, the lower lip is a distinct expression of the metabolic-limb pole, while the upper row of teeth represents the nerve-sense pole. Of the three metabolic functions (sucking, chewing and swallowing), sucking involves the lips and the cheeks, an elemental movement of affection, of pleasure. The opposite gesture of antipathy would be spitting. In the baby, sucking and swallowing are still one undivided function which are differentiate into two separate activities in the course of the first year. This separation is stimulated by taking in solid food.

Another differentiation in this area occurs in terms of the mouth being used for speaking. In the two babbling phases the infant gathers experiences enabling him to perceive and use the three zones separately.

The lip sounds **M**, **B**, **P** are rarely affected by disorders. The soul qualities connected with these sounds are: **M** — a gentle uniting of above and below, intensive pleasure (mmmh). **B** — firm enclosure (building, bed, boot, box). **P**: self-assertion and rejection (pah, pooh, pack up, poppycock).

Just like the crossing of the retina can be understood not only as giving spatial vision but also as being in contact with itself, and therefore a foundation of ego-experience in the body, likewise the experience of the lips as they constantly touch each other conveys an increased ego-experience. When someone presses their lips together, or bites on their lips, one recognizes increased concentration, pre-occupation with oneself, shame. A similar gesture is the covering of the mouth when one has to admit to a painful failure. In the same sense, an over-consciousness of the lips is equally unfavourable because it makes the person too strongly aware of themselves.

Disorders of the lip function

Two disorders in the realm of sucking and lip closure are to be mentioned here in particular. Weak and insufficient sucking in babies may lead to mouth breathing which is most unfavourable from a physiological point of view. The mucous membranes dry out which may lead to a taste disorder; moreover, there is often hypersalivation and slavering. Also the air breathed in is not cleansed, warmed and moistened as in normal nasal breathing. Consequently there is greater proneness to bronchitis and allergies.

Since air is breathed in more quickly, the breathing is less deep which may in turn lead to postural disorders. The typical picture of mentally disabled people with shoulders sloping forward, round back, tilted pelvis, limp knees as well as pes valgus and/or flat foot is an expression of this kind of general incarnation disorder.

Psychogenic mutisms, and elective mutism in particular, may also be counted among disorders of the lip quality in the broader sense. In this case, we do not just refer to the lips as such, but even more so to the related ability of the ego to set boundaries and open up. *Morphological (cleft lip face palate) and neurological (apoplexia) changes* may also affect the shape and function of the lips. As a result, the person affected is often very insecure, since the lips are closely related to the personality. Thus, people with facial nerve paralysis are often more affected by the change in facial expression than by the changed function. A weak or incorrect *use of the lip sounds* in adults also goes along with various other diseases and is therefore diagnostically and therapeutically relevant for the therapeutic speech practitioner. For instance, there is a connection between the lips and the sexual and excretory organs, which may be seized upon whenever there are disorders in these areas. This connection shows itself, for example, in related muscular structures of the orifices of the body, such as lips and anus (orbicular muscle), as well as the union of male and female form principles in the speech organs.

Thus, therapeutic speech has proved to be very effective with colitis (a severe diarrhoea) since it is not only able to exert a positive influence on the psychosomatic aspect of the disease (lack of boundaries) but also on the functional level.

From kinesiology it is well known that the *limp opening* of the mouth always leads to a generally weaker muscle tone in the body, as one can easily find out oneself by a simple arm test.

As already mentioned, genuine articulation disorders of the lip sounds are quite rare. However, weakness in the lips naturally leads to a weak articulation of those sounds.

Therapy and Prevention

As the previous reflections have shown, the child wants to 'love himself into the world.' In the beginning this love is expressed completely through the mouth. Therefore, prevention in this area means to return this love, *to breast-feed and care for* the child. Much has been said about the right time to wean the child. However, the recommendation to breast-feed as long as possible is neither to the advantage of the mother nor of the child. The natural maturation when the functions of sucking, chewing and swallowing are separated may be a natural limit, so that, as a rule, the child may be weaned by the end of the first year.

After this, the child also needs emotional and physical *closeness* which will transform into inner independence at the right time.

Where there is mouth breathing it is important to make sure that *the nose is free*, which may be a problem since these children tend to suffer from frequent colds. The very first and basic thing to do is to teach them how *to blow their nose* properly and often enough, that is to say through one nostril at a time while the other one is held closed. This simple and basic hygienic rule is often ignored and not passed on. *Smelling exercises* are also helpful, as well as closing the mouth consciously at times by holding a flat light object between the lips. Moreover *sucking and blowing games* of all kind — such as drinking through a straw — are suitable to strengthen the lip muscles.

Numerous other exercises are known in *myofunctional therapy.*[87]

Therapeutic speech works with verses and exercises made up mainly of lip sounds (**M, B, P, O, U**); the words should end on lip sounds, wherever possible.

Many of the speech exercises made by Rudolf Steiner are very suitable for this kind of training with older children (some of them from five years of age) and adults. Many popular children's verses also favour lip sounds. For instance: *Peter Peter Pumpkin Eater, One Misty Moisty Morning, Baa Baa Black Sheep.*

Just as the crossing of the visual axis not only mediates three-dimensional vision but may also be understood as 'touching oneself,' which is a basis of experiencing oneself as an ego in the body, the touching of the lips also means that one is constantly feeling oneself, which conveys a stronger sense of ego. Pressing one's lips together or biting one's lips is a sign of greater concentration, shame or self-absorption. A related gesture is to cover one's mouth when discovering an embarrassing lapse. In this sense 'over-awareness' of one's lips is also unfavourable since it makes one too self-conscious.

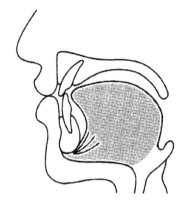

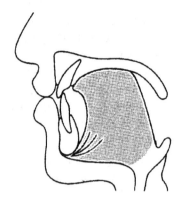

Figure 7 : Tongue in rest position

Figure 8: Diagram of a normal swallowing pattern

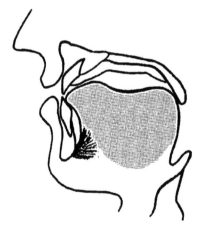

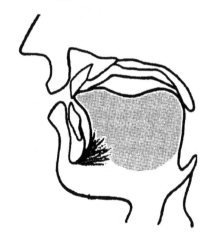

Figure 9 : Incorrect swallowing: pressure against the lower middle incisors

Figure 10: Incorrect swallowing: pressure against the upper incisors

From: Daniel Carliner: Myofunktionelle Therapie in der Praxis. Verlag Medizinisches Schrifttum, Mijnchen 1982.

Some authors have called the tongue the 'heart organ of the oral cavity.'[90] This supports the comparison of the fourfold structure of the tongue in its division into four muscular cords and the fourfold structure of the heart in its four chambers.

In any case, the dental region may be compared to the rhythmic system of the human being, since this is where the archetypal representatives of an upper pole (head, nerve-sense system, rest) and a lower pole (metabolic-limb system, movement) come together.

Disorders

The most frequent disorder of this area is a weak formative force of the upper pole of the human being. This may manifest itself as a developmental disorder in the form of a narrow position of the teeth in the upper jaw, *protrusion* of the front teeth due to tongue thrust, open bite due to thumb sucking, bottle feeding or incorrect placing of the tongue as well as *lisping* and incorrect *swallowing*.

According to therapeutic experience, this formative weakness appears more often in fair-haired children than in dark-haired ones. This phenomenon is due to the fact that in fair children the sulphurous, dissolving principle prevails over the formative principle, which is rich in iron.[91]

In the so-called 'incorrect swallowing,' i.e. swallowing with tongue thrust, the infantile pattern of swallowing has been retained beyond the first year. As already stated above, sucking and swallowing are not separated in babies. When swallowing, their tongue is thrust forward in their mouth.

In 'normal' swallowing, which the child acquires when taking in solid food, the tip of the tongue briefly presses against the point directly in the middle of the incisors, then moves the food on to the back of the oral cavity with a wave-like motion. From there it is passed on to the stomach by reflex action of the pharynx and oesophagus.

Since we swallow about two thousand times in twenty-four hours,[92] it is obvious that an incorrect swallowing motion applying pressure against the front teeth is likely to push the teeth forward. Nevertheless such deformities of the teeth often largely correct themselves in the first seven years, when healthy swallowing and breathing habits are developed.

A chronically open mouth favours the infantile pattern of swallowing enormously and should be improved first of all. The normally resting position of the tongue in the mouth is quite remarkable. It is not lying at the bottom of the mouth as might be expected due to its weight at rest, but is 'hanging' down from above in contact with the palate. Here, too, its love for movement is expressed beautifully by this lightness.

Each breath taken through the nose sucks the tongue gently up to the palate in this position due to the resulting vacuum in the back of the oral

cavity. The constant movement of the tongue against the palate in chewing and swallowing helps to widen the latter. This is also why the normal
function of the tongue is so important in order to created space in the
upper jaw for the second teeth.

When the rounding, arching forces of the head are even more impaired,
so that they are unable to assert themselves against the structuring force of
the lower pole which also forms the limbs, the *lip B jaw B palate B split*
(cleft lip and palate) results in the embryonic period. (Normally the palate
closes by the twelfth week of pregnancy.)

A milder form of the same tendency appears in the so-called *gothic
palate*, which often goes along with a narrow upper jaw and dysfunction
of the tongue. (From a dentist we heard about a child who, suffering brain
damage at the age of five months, gradually developed a gothic palate.)

Today the forces of the upper pole of the human being are getting
weaker at an alarming rate. During an examination of two hundred and
twenty-nine second-graders (seven and eight- year olds), 68% of the children were found to be mouth breathers, and a study of two hundred and
sixty-eight babies and infants at a clinic for outpatients in Erlangen,
Germany, found that only seventy of them were without disorders.

Out of the consonants S, Z, SH, L, N, D, T, rolled R, (lower lip and
upper row of teeth F and V), which may be affected by *dyslalia* , S and R
are the most difficult ones and therefore often incorrect.

The different types of lisp are also due to a weakness of the upper
organization. 'If the tongue goes beyond the teeth, it is the same as if the
soul were to entrust itself immediately to nature without a body,' said
Steiner, who characterized the normal articulation of the S as follows:
*'The lower and upper organisations of man, the organisations of head and
of limbs, are held in balance. The world has, so to speak, been captured
by man, he has it there within him; and now he on his part wants to send
forth his own being into the world without.* '[93] The correct S can be
achieved only by sufficient formative forces of the tongue, by an articulation that is neither hypo- nor hypertonic (strident lisp, frontal and/or inter-
dental lisp).

The rolled R, which gives a nice position and good sound to the
neighbouring vowels, is almost the polar opposite of the S, from the
point of view of the articulation. In order to roll the R the tip of the
tongue needs to be able to flutter loosely, while with the S it needs to
freeze, as it were, in the correct position. The sounds L, N, D, T are less
frequently subject to disorders but often even adults form these sounds
at the teeth. All of the consonants should be formed with the tip of the
tongue touching the LNDT-point which was already mentioned in connection with correct swallowing. Almost all dental sounds are formed

without the tongue directly touching the teeth. An exception is, for instance, the /**TH**/ in the English language. In the sense of this chapter the increasing differentiation of the German language, as expressed in the sound shifts, may be understood as an increasing differentiation of the elements of above and below, of form and movement. This also corresponds to an increasing formation of the astral body, which gives the impression that the German language is very ego-focused. In the English /**TH**/ and the articulation of **LNDT** at the teeth, these two principles are still interwoven.

The sound /**SH**/ is pronounced with the help of tongue and lips. This means that incorrect articulation may be due both to the position of the tongue and the lips (the lips need to be pushed forward in a pout). The sounds **F** and **V** in particular, which are formed with the help of the lower lip and the upper row of teeth, are to be seen in this context. *'And when we let lower lip and upper teeth work together in the right way in F and V, then what has been received by us from the whole sum of world secrets and is now wanting to come to expression finds that expression.'*[94] (In eurythmy the **F** expresses 'Know that I know.')

This leads us on to the fact that the dental region is assigned to *thinking*. If the level of thinking — of knowledge — is to be emphasized, the consonants of this particular area should be predominant in a speech. Therefore, in the sense of our description, grammatically incorrect or incomplete sentence construction *(dysgrammatism)* will also be assigned to a weakness or disorder of this area of the speech organs in a broader sense. 'Area of speech organs' here obviously means more than just the anatomical area but the whole functional connection of:

Dental Region → *Central Nervous System* → *Astral Body* → *Thinking*

The different types of aphasia, which may be the result of space-taking deformities or lesions, are also part of this functional context.

Therapeutic Approaches

Looking at this region in its functional context leads to certain therapeutic approaches. Here the interaction of all parts needs to be taken into consideration.

A clear articulation of the sounds of this area supports the maturation of the brain even when just listening to well articulated speech, and at the same time brings order into the astral body and thereby facilitates clear thinking. Clear thinking, on the other hand, schools the astral body, has a favourable effect on the brain and promotes a clear articulation. In both

is no more 'quality check' in the sense of the previous regions; any decision taken here is controlled by reflexes and may even surprise the person himself. All of these vital functions are action-oriented by nature, which is why this region is assigned to the will. It has a special connection to the whole body, to the limbs. Thus, articulating the K may quite naturally go along with stamping one's foot, while elemental emotions may be expressed by ha! hey! or ho! coming from the very back of the articulation area.

Since *chewing* has a lot to do with the will forces, it may be connected to this area. As already mentioned a few times, the ability to chew only really develops when the teeth push through; it may be regarded as a 'walking' activity of the speech organs. Well chewed food is obviously more easily digestible as well as easier to *taste* and to *swallow*.

Expressions such as 'they chewed it over' or 'she swallowed it' show that there is also an emotional connection to this region. 'Swallowed' here means 'accepted,' and the soul also should only swallow what was first chewed, that is to say thought through. What has been swallowed, then needs to be forgotten. There is no point to keep on wondering: was it the right decision?, etc. It is well known that undigested and unforgotten experiences may cause strain and depression.

The advantage of the soul's 'swallowing' is that it may be repeated. Just as only food that is well chewed and tasted is easily digestible, any experience needs to be digested consciously before it may be forgotten. The nightly review exercises recommended by Rudolf Steiner is very helpful in this context.[99]

The ability to close the larynx has an even greater influence on our physical strength than closing the lips. Thus, patients whose larynx has been removed by surgery are often hardly able to lift a chair. The resistance in the will area against the out-streaming air is missing. Likewise the articulatory force of **K**, **G** and **H** depends on the ability of the pharyngeal muscles and the vocal cords to give restraint as well as the support of the diaphragm.

Given the described closeness to the different vital functions, it is understandable why this region is assigned mainly to the *etheric body*. Its functions for the body are mainly at the level of sleeping consciousness which means that the person concerned is normally not aware of them.

However, the activity of the etheric body manifests itself above all in the liquid balance and the digestion of food. Thus, it is the etheric body which causes the constant production of saliva and the subsequent *swallowing*. This points to the fact that it is interconnected with the other bodily members (e.g. dry mouth when excited): the excited astral body (air body) brings the etheric functions to a halt — the mouth becomes dry.

Out of the sounds **Y**, **G**, **K**, **NG**, velar-**R** and **H**, the sounds **G** and **K** are acquired at a later stage of speech development and as such are often replaced with **D** and **T** by children. The will nature of these sounds is expressed in many words such as: good, grand, go, king, keeper, catastrophe etc. Linguistically speaking the **H**, the aspirate, is really nothing but a soft springboard for the vowel. The glottal stop as a hard vowel onset, is also to be mentioned in this context.

Disorders

From our point of view this includes first of all disorders of the functions of *chewing, swallowing* and of *the velum*; moreover, *stuttering, cluttering, nasality* and *incorrect articulation* of the velar sounds are to be included. The sound of the voice, insofar as it is formed by the hard and the soft palate, also represents a transition into this area.

The significance of *chewing* has already been mentioned. A frequent disorder of this function is the *grinding of one's teeth* (Bruxism).

It may be of psychogenic origin appearing mainly during sleep in people with unconscious tensions and problems. The person continues to 'chew' over their problems. A further origin of teeth grinding may be mal-occlusion of the jaws, which requires treatment by a dentist. *Functional swallowing disorders* were discussed in the previous chapter. Such disorders may also be symptoms of a cerebral disease (e.g. bulbar palsy), in which case, however, they tend to appear in connection with other symptoms.

In many people the function of the velum is quite unconscious. By way of a controlled opening or closing of the velum it is possible to produce intentional hyper- and denasality, which gives a strange sound to the voice. Hyporhinophonia occurs as a pathological phenomenon when the nose is more or less blocked due to inflammation or when children have enlarged tonsils. Hyperrhinophonia is mainly due to paralysis of the velum, from different origins, or cleft palate.

On the whole, we may describe the flow of speech as a leading out of the formed stream of breath, as will gesture in the breath stream. *Stuttering* and *cluttering* are interruptions of the stream of breath. This helps to make a first assignment of this disorder to the velar region, the will region. In spontaneous speaking this gesture is structured and restrained by the form of the speech and the articulation — both of which are conscious activities.

An uninhibited yell as an emotional will expression is least restrained, while the expression of complicated thoughts is naturally structured by pauses. Words and sentences that are difficult to articulate challenge the skills of the speaker and may occasionally cause stumbling over the articulation.

Therefore, it is particularly informative to look at the will gesture of the flow of speech according to its relationship to thinking and willing. Stuttering means that too much influence is being exerted on this flow by the nervous-sense system, while in cluttering there is a one-sided predominance of the will activity. In cluttering the speech impulse partly overpowers the faculties of the upper pole: articulation and thinking. The stutterer, on the other hand, blocks his speech impulse by too much thinking (negative expectations, searching for alternative words) and automatically misarticulates (clonic or tonic cramps). Following the description of the two types of constitution given in Chapter 9 on neurasthenia and hysteria, the symptom of cluttering might be assigned to the hysteric constitution, while the symptom of stuttering belongs to the neurasthenic constitution.

The speech impulse as formed breath is interfered with by any impulse inhibiting this stream of joyful communication from outside. Animosity and overcorrectness in the environment and/or fear rising up from inside will lead to overemphasizing the inhalation or to holding the breath completely, as anybody knows from moments of shock.

In stuttering this type of breathing is intensified up to speaking on the inhalation, or the speech is pushed out with the remaining air after silent exhalation.

As far as the equilibrium of vowels and consonants is concerned, the consonantal element is predominant in stuttering — above all the impact sounds, which anyway slow the breath down. The vowels, which mediate the feeling, as well as the breath, are the ones to suffer. This explains why most stutterers are able to sing without problems, since in singing the consonants recede in favour of voice and breath.

Stuttering is often described as an unsuitable attempt at re-establishing fluency. In many cases it goes along with convulsive secondary symptoms (such as movements of head and limbs, distortions of the face, convulsions etc.) In cramps the harmonious interweaving of etheric body and astral body, which makes our movements smooth, is interfered with by an excessive activity of the astral body. This means that the physical body temporarily predominates in the muscles concerned, which manifests itself in convulsive movements and hardening. Moreover, one's self-perception — mediated by the ego-organization — is disturbed because the astral body predominates in the form of negative feelings.

In the soul this manifests itself as fear. Fear of speaking, fear of expectations, avoidance of difficult words and situations, a poor self-image and poor self-perception — all of this leads to the described impediments of the will expression of speech. Since the emotional background is so charged in stutterers, imprinting itself, as a long-term disorder, into the etheric body as a bad habit, a relapse is likely to occur even after longer periods of improvement (remission). Teaching the patient to take such relapses with equanimity is the foundation of any promising therapy.

Therapeutic Approaches

Based on the insights just described, therapeutic speech has something to offer which mainstream stutter therapy does not have: artistic elements. Since stuttering leaves an imprint in the etheric body, and since the flow of speech, on the whole, is an unconscious process, any therapeutic intervention has to aim for long-term effects. In the following, individual elements from the overall concept will be described.

Positive experiences of almost stutter-free speaking

All stutterers are able to speak fluently under guidance. This experience is essential, especially at the beginning of a therapy. Most stutterers will fluently repeat a poem or a rhythmical text after the therapist, thereby practising a harmonious balance between inhalation and exhalation. With the right length of line and the right balance and with the appropriate practice a deep influence can be exerted on the breathing. Lines made up of more than three feet are dominated by the breath and prove to be particularly favourable. Of the Greek metres the anapaest and the dactyl are most suitable — the latter mainly embedded in the hexameter. They can be used either to stimulate or to calm down and harmonize the relationship of breath, voice and articulation. The trochee or more specific rhythms, such as the choriambus, are suitable as well. To lengthen the breath these rhythms can be used in specific verses. The following two examples are from working with children.

> *Immer ruhig geht das Denken,*
> *Denken fliesset ohne Absatz nur dahin.*
> *Hin so fliesset auch mein Sprechen wie ein Strom.*
> *Strom, der über keines Felsens scharfe Kante bricht.*

> *Slowly, calmly flows our thinking,*
> *Thinking flowing unimpeded onwards.*
> *On should also flow my speech like gentle waters,*
> *Waters which no craggy boulder's rocky edges breaks.*

know about stuttering.' Wendlandt's book is not written from an anthro-posophical point of view but is highly recommended for the fundamental information it gives.[101] Alfred Baur has written a stimulating book on stut-tering children from an anthroposophical perspective.[102]

12.4 Voice and Breath

Below the *velar region* is the *larynx*. It is the last closure before the bronchi and the lungs. Unlike the lips the vocal chords are turned inside looking whitish, instead of red (which means that they are hardly supplied with blood). To produce the tone the vocal chords begin to vibrate, and these vibrations are further processed by the vocal tract and the speech instrument. Even for purely anatomic reasons this way of creating *speech* is possible only for human beings, since only the human oropharynx is spacious enough. In all mammals (including the primates) the larynx is elevated as in the human infant. Only when the larynx moves down is it possible for the voice to form the vowels by connecting the larynx to the oral cavity in the appropriate way.

As already mentioned, the velar region is the boundary between con-scious and unconscious functions. In the healthy process of speaking and singing the functions of the larynx should not become conscious. Only in the oral region does the possibility for conscious sound formation begin which is further differentiated by the tongue and the lips.

The breath has already been discussed in detail elsewhere in this book.

Voice Disorders

A large number of functional disorders of the voice are caused by an unphysiological use of and an increased awareness of the larynx (hyper-functional dysphonia). Due to various reasons, the articulation activity of lips, tongue and palate becomes weaker, immediately causing a greater strain on the voice. The cause of this is often: 1) *tiredness or general exhaustion*; 2) *a constant overstraining because one is pulled out too much* (teacher). This means that the upper pole of the human being loses its centre and is weakened. Weakness of the upper pole in a neurasthenic constitution causes shallow breathing, which in turn is unphysiological for the use of the voice (lack of support).

Hypofunctional symptoms often turn into hyperfunction. Likewise there may be hypofunctional exhaustion with hyperfunction. This 'aim-less' activity, as it were, of the astral body is characteristic of a state of exhaustion. The astral body is no longer able to create a healthy tension

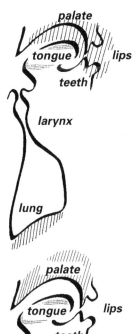

Figure 11: Normal articulation and voice: Consciousness of articulation and voice

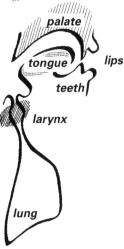

Figure 12: Hyperfuctional Dysphonia: Incorrect Consciousness in region of larynx (tension).

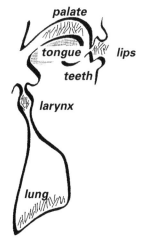

Figure 13: Hypofunctional Dysphonia: Consciousness (tension) wanders weak and unpurposefully here and there.

between the polarities of diaphragm and frontal speech instruments and consequently swings back and forth between taking hold of the body too strongly or not at all. It is not possible in this context to include more specific *diseases of the larynx*.

Breathing Disorders

Vegetative, unconscious spontaneous breathing is distinctly different from breathing in connection with speaking and singing. One main difference is the longer exhalation in speaking and singing.

Apart from organic restrictions caused by accidents or diseases, disorders of the spontaneous respiration will mostly be *functional*. In our civilization only few adults show a really healthy spontaneous breathing (see also Chapter 7, 'General Diagnosis in Therapeutic Speech'). Describing the subtle deviations of the breath from what is healthy would go beyond the scope of this exposition, unless mentioned in connection with individual diseases. Just three examples worth mentioning here are: s*hallow breathing*, a much *decelerated breathing* and *hyperventilation*. While the latter two cause a shift in the ratio of pulse and breath, all three are both cause and expression of functional disorders.

In various other chapters of this book there are further references to subtle breathing disorders accompanying all diseases.[103]

Therapeutic Approaches

Since the whole of this book deals with the subject of voice and breathing therapy, in different connections, this subject is only to be touched upon here. Therapeutic speech starts with articulation and breathing exercises, finally treating the voice itself with *vowel exercises*, according to the particular disorder. This leads regularly to positive results, since with regard to the voice in particular nothing can be achieved without artistic feeling.

Depending on whether the disorder needs to be treated more in the area of the pharynx and larynx or whether it is caused by an incorrect articulation activity, the therapy will focus on the vowels /**a**/, /**e**/, /**i**/ or /**o**/, /**u**/, /**ü**/, respectively. The so-called '*Aale*' exercise is an instrument for a universal long-term treatment and optimization of the functions of the voice; the principles underlying the exercise may be adjusted to the individual case.

Treating voice problems very often involves shifting the patient's attention and vocal activity forward to the *instrument of articulation* and downward to the *diaphragmatic support* in order to create a free space in the middle (chest and larynx) with no interfering waking consciousness.

In the context of anthroposophical medicine, breathing therapy is

The therapist will also notice possible morphological deviations of the speech instrument that may cause articulation disorders. An unclear, hasty formation of the sounds or an overprecise articulation gives the therapist basic information about the patient, as does the position of his voice and its resonance spaces in the sinuses, the larynx and the chest. The voice can tell the therapist something about the soul of the patient, about where it tends to withdraw or to unfold itself freely. The voice may be light or dark, warm or cold, monotonous, lively, hard, soft, timid, energetic, loud, quiet, cracked, hoarse or clear, revealing the mood of the soul and painting a clear picture of the person's individuality and constitution. An ordinary conversation may reveal certain breathing habits, that is to say the tendency, for instance, to let go of the breath or to hold it back, to take quick shallow breaths or to speak with too much breath.

If the therapist manages from the start to open up to the patient in such a way that he can feel the patient's habits of articulating, speaking and breathing in his own body,[106] to reenact, as it were, in his own rhythmic system the way the patient is incarnated — an experience which then needs to be deepened again and again in the course of the therapy — he can get a first idea of whether the person is happy or reluctant to enter the therapeutic process. For 'in the speech everything is expressed with absolute certainty.'[107]

By opening up fully to the patient's speech, the therapist can make the patient feel that he is entering on a path of self-development and self-healing which will enable him to shed one-sided habits that make him ill. Giving an introduction (short but geared to the individual) into the way health, speech and breathing are interrelated the therapist can often help the patient in the very first meeting to create a happy anticipation of the therapeutic process. If the therapist shows that he can accompany the patient inwardly, the patient feels that he is being understood and accepted. The initial question: why should I do therapeutic speech when I can speak well, changes into interested amazement when the patient realizes how interrelated the human being is with his speech. This is something that *every* human being can experience immediately, no matter what his background is. For this connects to something everyone is familiar with and can use all the time: one's speech.

2. Support Phase

This very feeling of being understood and accepted in one's speech is then deepened in the artistic process. At the same time speech habits that may have prevailed for years are broken, which may cause a temporary feeling of insecurity. But like any change of habit this is an extra call upon the ego to be present. The patient learns to listen to himself and to the speech practitioner in a completely new way — namely not to the content of what is being said, but to speech itself, to the sounds. The speaker's innermost being is expressed and looked at, which leads to the experience: I am the way I speak, but at the same time my speech contains the seeds, the potential to become what I am not yet.

No matter how ill the patient may be or how difficult his life may be, the therapist can always make him understand that simply by possessing the ability to speak, something complete and healing is constantly working in him in a creative way and that the spiritual entity living in him is eternal and indestructible. Therefore, when the patient first begins he should not be made aware of what is disturbed in his way of speaking and breathing, but of all the things he can do, of how hundreds of muscles move to form a sound, of how his voice sounds and is carried by the air.

All initial exercises should be aimed at making the patient aware of his speech instrument and its articulating activity. This way of experiencing one's physical body in a creative, artistic way makes the person incarnate more deeply.

The patient begins to experience how each sound in all the languages of the world tends to focus the human being on forming a middle. Then, how the stream of voice and breath is led forth from the middle of the mouth, with each inhalation bringing the soul into the sound formation in order to release it again on the formed exhalation once it has taken hold of the body and worked it through in the right way.

Feeling joy in the smallest, seemingly most ordinary sound experience and in the creative speech process which is now seized consciously will immediately deepen the breath. This joy should never wane, no matter how intensely one is working on a problem, for the joy of speaking is the greatest healing factor in this therapy.[108] Since the patient speaks the exercises and texts after the therapist in the beginning, he need not worry about himself and his problems for the moment but can feel supported and enveloped by the therapist's speech, which will build him up and carry him also by listening to it.

Only when the patient has found support in his own speech by thus listening and speaking after the therapist can the next step be taken in a healing way: to break up one's old habits.

3. Phase of Conscious Confrontation

The patient is now faced with the challenge to change his previous unconscious way of speaking, overcome his *inherited speech* and find that speech which is in accordance with and beneficial to himself and his breathing.

Step by step he approaches the speech laws which are already contained in the first five articulation exercises. He learns to enter consciously into the sounds, which until now were formed unconsciously, and to follow the stream of breath into the air. He leads the breath downward, deepening it rhythmically, giving support to his voice by shaping the consonants. In this phase of the therapy, the transition from the habitual to the new way of speaking may be experienced by the patient as a painful process of looking at himself. The old habits do not carry him any more, and new ones have not yet been fully developed. Becoming sensitive to one's own one-sidedness and weaknesses may cause temporary irritation which may be an impediment to the previously instinctive flow of speech.

The speech movements which are now made conscious will be halted, and the former spontaneity of the speech process will be interrupted temporarily in order to be later regained at a higher level. This slight state of uncertainty requires the patient to make a renewed decision to work on himself and his set, one-sided speech habits. It will be necessary to encourage him continuously and give him clear instructions as to what and how to practise. The support which the patient could find in the therapist's speech in the beginning of the therapy process can now be found partly in his own voice and breath. This will be a basis for any further steps he takes in practising.

At this stage the therapy can become very intensive since the patient is confronted on all sides with the expectation to change, and he has to make an increased will effort.

He experiences increasingly that the cause of his disease, on the one hand, and his speech and breathing patterns, on the other, are one and the same, and he may be reluctant to take the decisive step of change. In general, this is the moment when the breathing deepens and a new connection has been made between speech and body movements. The skills that have already been acquired are in danger of becoming automatic again, that is to say of being used without ego presence. Therefore the therapist will need a lot of imagination and patience to keep the ego of the patient interested so that it stays present in the speech process. What is particularly helpful is to find ever new pictures for the exercises, some of which the patient knows already. Working more with rhythms at this stage helps to relax the patient and disperse paralysing self-doubt.

4. Phase of Maturation of the Self

This phase also is characterized by a transition to new processes of movement, speech and breathing. But, in general, at this stage of the therapy there are no deep crises any more. Gait, posture, look and facial expression of the patient have all changed, which is often noticed by the doctor as well. Family and close friends of the patient often say that the way he speaks has changed also, and has become freer. This encourages the patient to keep going. Often a certain degree of healing is experienced so that he stops taking his medicine or seeing the doctor. Even if this means that the healing forces inherent in the speech are beginning to work, the patient must not overestimate his own abilities at this point. The new skills must be practised again and again so that they can be effective even at times of crisis or relapse. They have to become a habit. Daily speech practice has become part of the patient's life, also affecting his rhythmical processes.

What is particularly important is for the patient to hear how his speech must sound in order to have a healing effect on his organism. He is able to listen to his own speech, to correct himself and thus keep striving independently for the ideal. After the physical prerequisites for the patient's healing have been improved with the help of articulation and rhythmic exercises, his soul may now be stimulated to perceive, for instance, the dynamic inherent in the speech and gain strength from it.

5. Phase of Self-Orientation

Not all patients achieve this phase and the following two. Often previous phases must be repeated, or phase five is reached with regard to certain exercises only.

The patient increasingly realizes and accepts that the path of therapy offers individual help for his life. He has found certain constitutional exercises he can identify with. He is able to use a speech exercise effectively whenever necessary; for instance, to change his breathing pattern when he is in respiratory distress by speaking a hexameter in a rhythmic way, or use an exercise to expand his breathing when he has a panic attack. Some exercises are used purposefully like a medicine that strengthens, invigorates, calms down or takes away pain. This phase often goes along with biographical changes.

By identifying more and more with his speech the patient develops new confidence in himself. This may also give new meaning to his life. Just as the old speech habits have been cast off like an old garment, the individual may strive to break free from static living patterns, to question his previous way of life and start looking for new aims. Here the placement exercises, which bring clarity to thinking, feeling and willing, may give a certain help.

At this stage many patients wish to talk with the therapist; they wish to see and understand the connection between what they have acquired so far and their everyday life. Clearly a new relationship between ego speech, thereby re-establishing his health as far as possible, the therapist faces a more comprehensive task. He has to clearly analyse the quality of his own bodies and initiate positive change.

First of all, he has to change his own habits of speaking and breathing, which is possible only by working untiringly with the speech exercises. By learning to listen to oneself from outside, as it were, a process of detaching from one's own subjective personality begins.

The sounds and sound sequences practised ever and again gradually change the student's speech habits, making him more sensitive to the laws of speech. An unconscious, mechanical articulation is increasingly replaced by the word shaped consciously and actively by the speech instrument.

Practising also prevents the therapist from being influenced too much by the patient, and the other way round. Being schooled by the sounds, the soul forces of thinking, feeling and willing become ever more conscious and are increasingly influenced and directed by the ego. Gradually it becomes possible to tell which part of the personality stands in the way of a healthy speech and breathing process.

The therapist must consciously leave behind his own intellectual ideas, his subjective feeling and the desire to assert his own will. With the help of the consonants he can learn to objectify his own will activity by translating sound *idea* into sound *movement.*

The right way of working with the vowels and the training of the voice that goes along with it results in a more sober attitude towards one's own feelings. It is necessary to ask oneself continually to what extent there is self-pleasure and sentimentality in one's voice, which should be warm and ensouled but free from subjective emotions.

Making the breath step along with the speech (as in the syllable step or the rhythm) strengthens and clarifies the will, making one's speech ever more fluent. In this way the therapist trains himself with the help of the speech to become ever more objective in the way he looks at the patient and his disease, to leave behind sympathy and antipathy and to stop acting from his subjective will, but instead to go by what the patient needs for his healing. While his personality has to make certain sacrifices, his individuality will increasingly unfold.

This really means that the therapist becomes a student who often owes the progress of his development to the person with whom he is doing therapy.

This process is something to be aimed for by continuous practice. Like with anything alive, it is not static but there is constant movement and change. Thus, by overcoming what is too personal, a part of the soul may become one with the speech, so that the ego may develop and practise thinking, feeling and willing with the help of the speech. In the rhythmical breathing process formed by the sounds, the ego-consciousness can take hold of the ego-force.[111] The person schooling himself in this way will repeatedly come up against the limitations of his own personality and constitution. By bravely trying to overcome the crises of their own process of individualization they will be able to have a strengthening and invigorating effect on the ego of the patient blurred by the disease.

To the extent that the ego is able to overcome the boundaries of the body, the person begins to be a vessel for the spiritual forces immanent in the speech from the sphere where the healing impulses may be received and passed on. This sphere is also where poetry originates, which the speech forms out of the connection of soul and spirit, not according to the needs of the body, as is the rule in everyday life. This means that true poetry nourishes and heals the soul. On his schooling path, the therapist can experience poetry as a source of joy and confidence that will never run dry. He can learn to put into pictures what he hears in the patient's speech and from these pictures find the right therapeutic process. Any further steps along this schooling path are really part of a future aim of humanity.

Any change brought about in the speech instrument, the breathing and the voice will affect the whole human organism. By continually penetrating the physical formative forces of speech with spirit and soul the healing forces in every human being are strengthened. In this sense, it is understandable that regular speech practice will harmonize the ratio of pulse and breathing. The more light processes, that is to say spirituality, the human being takes in via the breath, the healthier he will be in the future and the more it will be possible to bring about healing through the word.[112]

Endnotes

1 Vgl. Böhme, Gerhard, *Sprach-, Sprech-, Stimm- und Schluckstörungen*, Volume 1, pp. 1-7.

2 See Bibliography.

3 Report from the conference 'Adäquate Forschungsmethoden für die Therapeutische Sprachgestaltung.' Herdecke, 1998.

4 GA 282, *Speech and Drama*, lecture of Sep 21, 1924.

5 *Ibid,* lecture of Sep 22, 1924.

6 From a notebook from Rudolf Steiner.

7 GA 281, *Speech and the Art of Poetry*, lecture of March 29, 1923.

8 GA 280, *Creative Speech*.

9 GA 282, *Speech and Drama*, lecture of Sep 5, 1924.

10 GA 279, *Eurythmy as Visible Speech*, lecture of June 24, 1924.

11 GA 110, *Anthroposophical Spiritual Science and Medical Therapy*, lecture of April 17, 1921.

12 GA 251, *Cosmic Workings in Earth and Man*, lecture of Oct 27, 1923.

13 GA 315, *Curative Eurythmy*, lecture of April 13, 1921.

14 GA 280, *Creative Speech*, 'Course on the Art of Speech Formation,' 1922, dictation by Marie Steiner.

15 *Ibid.*

16 Schöpen, H., *Psychiatrie der Gegenwart*, Volume 1.

17 See Endnote 4.

18 GA 348, *From Comets to Cocaine*, lecture of Dec 27, 1922.

19 *Ibid,* lecture of Feb 3, 1923.

20 GA 212, *The Human Soul in Relation to World Evolution,* lecture of May 26, 1922.

21 See also the chapter General Diagnosis in Therapeutic Speech.

22 GA 21, *Von Seelenrätseln,* in 'Die physischen und die geistigen Abhängigkeiten der Menschen-Wesenheit' out of 'Skizzenhaften Erweiterungen zum Inhalt dieser Schrift.'

23 See in addition the lectures in *Foundations of Human Experience,* especially the lecture of Sep 1, 1919, GA 293; also Vogel, Lothar, *Der dreigliedrige Mensch, Morphologische Grundlage einer allgemeinen Menschenkunde.*

24 See also the chapter Typical Speech Disorders, their Assignment to the Articulation Regions and Therapy.

25 Hanmann, Johann Georg, *Schriften zur Sprache*.

26 See also the Figures 7–10 in the chapter Typical Speech Disorders, their Assignment to the Articulation Regions and Therapy.

27 GA 9, *Theosophy.* An introduction to the Supersenible Knowledge of the world and the destination of Man.

28 See the table in the lecture of Sep 21, 1924, in *Speech and Drama,* GA 282.

29 Lowndes, Florin, *Das Erwecken des Herzdenkens. Wesen und Leben des sinnlichkeitsfreien Denkens in der Darstellung Rudolf Steiners*, Stuttgart 1998.

30 See Endnote 4.

31 GA 127, Anthroposophical Quarterly, Vol. 21, No.4, lecture of Feb 25, 1911.

32 GA 127. See also the chapter General Diagnosis in Therapeutic Speech.

33 GA 222, *The Driving Force of Spiritual Powers in World History,* lecture of March 11, 1923.

Bibliography

Altmier, Marianne, *Der kunsttherapeutische Prozess*. Stuttgart, 1995.

Baur, Alfred, *Fließend sprechen*. Novalis, Schaffhausen, 1988.

— *Healing Sounds: Fundamentals of Chirophonetics*. Rudolf Steiner College, Fair Oaks, CA, 1993.

Bigenzahn, W., *Orofaziale Dysfunktionen*. Thieme, Stuttgart, 1998.

Böhme, Gerhard, *Sprach-, Sprech-, Stimm- und Schluckstörungen*. Stuttgart 1997.

Degenaar, G. (Ed.), *Krankheitsfälle und andere medizinische Fragen, besprochen mit Rudolf Steiner*. Manuskriptdruck, no date.

Denjean-von Stryk, Barbara, *Sprich, dass ich dich sehe*. Freies Geistesleben, Stuttgart, 1983.

Dreher, Wera, *Studien und Übungen zur Sprachtherapie*. Freies Geistesleben, Stuttgart, 1983.

Duwan, Ilja, *Sprachgestaltung und Schauspielkunst. Vom Kunstimpuls Marie Steiner. Übungen für Lautstimmungen und dramatische Gebärden*. Goetheanum, Dornach, 1990.

Elsner, E., *Raumfahrt in Stichworten*. Kiel, 1973.

Fiechter, Hans Paul, *Grundlagen einer praktischen Poetik*. Freies Geistesleben, Stuttgart, 1996.

Friedrich, G. and Bigenzahn, W., *Phoniatrie*. Hans Huber, Bern 1995.

Garliner, Daniel., *Myofunctional Therapy*. W.B. Saunders Company, 1981.

Hamann, Johann Georg, *Schriften zur Sprache*.

Healy, Jane M., *Endangered minds: Why our children don't think*. Touchstone Press, 1991.

Heide, Paul von der, *Therapie mit geistig-seelischen Mitteln. Kunsttherapie, Psychotherapie, Psychosomatik*. Goetheanum, Dornach, 1997.

Herberg, Ursula, *A New Approach to Speech Therapy*. Manuscript , 1993.

Husemann, Armin J., *Der Zahnwechsel des Kindes. Ein Spiegel seiner seelischen Entwicklung*. Goetheanum, Dornach, 1996.

Jakobson, Roman, *Kindersprache, Aphasie und allgemeine Lautgesetze*. Suhrkamp, Frankfurt.

Koepke, Hermann, *Das neunte Lebensjahr. Seine Bedeutung in der Entwicklung des Kindes*. Goetheanum, Dornach, 1997.

König, Karl, *The First Three Years*. Floris Books, Edinburgh, 2004.

König, Karl; Arnim, Georg von; Herberg, Ursula, *Sprachverständnis und Sprachbehandlung*. Freies Geistesleben, Stuttgart, 1978.

Kralik, Jörg von, *Sprachgestaltung und dramatische Darstellungskunst.* Goetheanum, Dornach, 1984.

Lorenz-Poschmann, Agathe, *Die Sprachwerkzeuge und ihre Laute.* Goetheanum, Dornach, 1983.

— *Therapie durch Sprachgestaltung.* Goetheanum, Dornach, 1983.

Lowndes, Florin, *Das Erwecken des Herzdenkens. Wesen und Leben des sinnlichkeitsfreien Denkens in der Darstellung Rudolf Steiners. Umriss einer Methodik.* Freies Geistesleben, Stuttgart, 1998.

Lutzker, Peter, *Der Sprachsinn.* Freies Geistesleben, Stuttgart, 1996.

Martens, Martin Georg, *Rhythmen der Sprache.* Goetheanum, Dornach, 1976.

Müller, Heinz, *Healing Forces in the Word and its Rhythms.* Rudolf Steiner Schools Fellowship Publications, Forest Row, 1983.

Schöpen, *Psychiatrie der Gegenwart.* Mannheim.

Slezak-Schindler, Christa, *Der Schulungsweg der Sprachgestaltung und praktische Anregungen für die sprachkünstlerische Therapie.* Goetheanum, Dornach, 1994.

— *Künstlerisches Sprechen im Schulalter.* Pädagogische Forschungsstelle beim Bund der freien Waldorfschulen. Stuttgart, 1978.

— *Sprüche und Lautspiele.* Self published, Stuttgart, 1984.

— *Vom Leben mit dem Wort. Fünf heilende Wirksamkeiten der Sprache und des Sprechens.* Goetheanum, Dornach, 1992.

Steiner, Rudolf, Complete Edition *(Gesamtausgabe, GA)* in Rudolf Steiner Verlag, Dornach.

Stockmeyer, E.A. Karl, *Rudolf Steiner's Curriculum for Waldorf Schools.*

Riper, Charles van, *The Treatment of Stuttering.* Prentice Hall, 1973.

Vogel, Lothar, *Der dreigliedrige Mensch, Morphologische Grundlage einer allgemeinen Menschenkunde.* Goetheanum, Dornach, 1992.

Wendlandt, Wolfgang, *Sprachstörungen im Kindesalter.* Thieme, Stuttgart, 1998.

— *Zum Beispiel Stottern.* Pfeiffer, 1984.

— *Stottern ins Rollen bringen.* Bundesvereinigung Stotterer-Selbsthilfe e.V., 1994.

Wulff, Henning, *Diagnose von Sprach- und Stimmstörungen.* Ernst Reinhardt, 1983.

Zinke, Johanna, *Luftlautformen sichtbar gemacht. Sprache als plastische Gestaltung der Luft.* Freies Geistesleben, Stuttgart, 2000.

Research

Recent research has been exploring the effects of Anthroposophical Therapeutic Speech (ATS) on heart rate variability, oscillations of heart rate and respiratory synchronization, and heart rate rhythmicity and cardiorespiratory coordination. While it is beyond the scope of this book to report the full findings of this research, the interested reader will find the published research papers in the following journals:

• Bettermann, Henrik; von Bonin, Dietrich; Frühwirth, Matthias; Cysarz, Dirk; Moser, Maximilian. 'Effects of speech therapy with poetry on heart rate rythmicity and cardiorespiratory coordination'. International Journal of Cardiology, Vol. 84:77–88, 2002.

• Cysarz, Dirk; von Bonin, Dietrich; Lackner, Helmut; Heusser, Peter; Moser, Maximilian; Bettermann, Henrik. 'Oscillations of heart rate and respiration synchronize during poetry recitation'. *American Journal of Physiology, Heart Circulation Physiology*, Vol. 287:H579–H587, 2004.

Useful Organisations

Association for Anthroposophic Speech Arts in North America
www.creativespeech.org

International Coordination of Anthroposophic Art Therapies
www.icaat-medsektion.net

Association of Anthroposophic Therapeutic Arts
www.aata-uk.org

Ears and Hearing (formally tested?)

ENT results:

3) Speech:
a) Impulse for speech

b) Breathing, flow of speech (fluency), stuttering etc.:

c) Balance of flowing and formative elements in the child's speech:

d) Balance of vowels, quality of voice, modulation, ability to sing in tune, vocal range, singing:

e) Balance of consonants, articulation placements in speech organ (e.g. lisp), sound groups, difference between spontaneous speaking and speaking after therapist:

f) Individual sounds:

lips		*tongue/teeth*	*palate*	
MBP	*FV*	*LNDT SZR SH CH J*	*YGK CH (loch) HR*	
				normal
				limited
				missing

g) Nasality:

4) Language and thinking:
a) Repetition of language, sense of word, short term memory (in number of syllables):

b) Vocabulary (active and passive):

c) Understanding, sense of thought, forming of concepts:

d) Sentence construction, including grammar, complexity of sentences and Mean Length of Utterance, 3 levels according to König: saying, naming, talking

e) Academic skills:

f) Reading and writing:

g) Non-verbal performance:

h) Pragmatic Language Skills, use of social language, answers and poses questions appropriately

5) General characteristics: habits, quirks etc.

6) Past Interventions: early years education, speech and language therapy, developmental issues:

7) Summary:

8) Recommendations:

_____

Evaluator/ ATS Therapist

Index

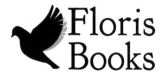
Floris
Books

For news on all our **latest books,**
and to receive **exclusive discounts,**
join our mailing list at:

florisbooks.co.uk

Plus subscribers get a FREE book
with every online order!

We will never pass your details to anyone else.